The Pearlescent Flame

The Pearlescent Flame

LIVING BEAUTIFUL

JESSICA
PUCKETT,
MS, L.Ac.

Writers of the Round Table Press
PO Box 511, Highland Park, IL 60035
www.roundtablecompanies.com

Publisher and Executive Editor: Corey Michael Blake
Editor: Katie Gutierrez
Creative Director, Post Production, Digital Publishing: David Charles Cohen
Directoress of Happiness: Erin Cohen
Director of Author Services: Kristin Westberg
Facts Keeper: Mike Winicour
Front Cover Design: Karla Oroz Puckett
Interior Design and Layout, Back Cover: Sunny DiMartino
Proofreading: Rita Hess
Last Looks: Jess Place
Digital Book Conversion: Sunny DiMartino

Printed in the United States of America
First Edition: March 2013

Library of Congress Cataloging-in-Publication Data
Puckett, Jessica
The Pearlescent flame: living beautiful / Jessica Puckett; edited by Katie
Gutierrez.—1st ed. p. cm.
ISBN 978-1-939418-13-5
Library of Congress Control Number: 2013934437

RTC Publishing is an imprint of Writers of the Round Table, Inc.
Writers of the Round Table Press and the RTC Publishing logo
are trademarks of Writers of the Round Table, Inc.

To BKH, *the most beautiful.*

CONTENTS

xi . . . . ACKNOWLEDGMENTS

xiii . . . . INTRODUCTION: Alchemy and Living Beautiful

CHAPTER 1

1 . . . . Red Flame: Hometown

CHAPTER 2

13 . . . . Orange Flame: Paris

CHAPTER 3

35 . . . . Yellow Flame: New Orleans

CHAPTER 4

55 . . . . Green Flame: Hebrides Islands

CHAPTER 5

73 . . . . Blue Flame: Colorado

CHAPTER 6

91 .... Violet Flame: Chicago

CHAPTER 7

109 .... Silver Flame

CHAPTER 8

121 .... Gold Flame: Chicago

CHAPTER 9

131 .... Pearlescent Flame: New Orleans

149 .... ABOUT JESSICA PUCKETT

ACKNOWLEDGMENTS

So many amazing riders accompanied me on this roller coaster journey. Thanks to those who were willing to sit with me in the front car, hands up and screaming as we tipped over the edge of the hill, looking straight ahead at the unobstructed view. Thank you to those who were willing to ride but wanted to be strapped safely in the middle—you kept me grounded. Finally, to my back seat riders: the true enthusiasts. I love you. You were there, not knowing where we were going but trusting the path, whipping through the air while being tossed side to side, knowing it was a risk but seeking the thrill. All of you inspire me.

Alchemy and Living Beautiful

ALCHEMY: *a power or process of transmuting something common into something special.*

TRANSMUTATION: *to change or alter in form, appearance, or nature and especially to a higher form.*

Little girls want to be beautiful. They dress up, slip into their mothers' high heels, and live in a world of make-believe. In secret daydreams, they imagine being surrounded by people who appreciate their unique beauty—or, at least, I did.

With flaming red hair, big brown eyes, and pale skin, I did not resemble the typical Southern girl . . . and the typical ones around me never let me forget it. While the girls I knew at school spent their summers lying by the pool, slathering their bodies with oil, I hid from the sun for fear of multiplying my freckles and developing skin cancer.

My grandmother was my beauty champion. She was an independent, strong woman who didn't need a man (though she was married for sixty-five years). She told me my red hair made me special. As for the pale, almost translucent skin, she said, "Honey, back in the day that meant you were a part of the high society." With no use for self-pity, she had a convincing way of reassuring me of my beauty and worth as a woman.

Even with my grandmother's voice in my head, it took thirty years for me to embrace my own beauty—and understand what "living beautiful" meant. I had to accept that the only thing I could control in the world was myself; I could not change any hardship, heartbreak, or people's opinions—only my reactions to them. So, I made a choice to transform myself and the way I viewed the world. This was not only for my benefit but also for my daughter, who deserves a mother who is not afraid to live her authentic life.

In keeping with this new journey, I turned down entry to medical school in 2003 and decided to enroll in a graduate program for Oriental Medicine. Becoming an acupuncturist was not something I could have anticipated, but that path gave me the tools I needed to understand true beauty.

As a pre-med undergraduate, I was required to learn the history of chemistry. I happen to love history, particularly ancient European history, and the subject immediately caught my interest. I decided to study a semester abroad during my first year of college and was drawn to the old apothecaries of Europe. It seemed I couldn't get away from the evolution of chemistry—and it all started with alchemy.

Alchemy is the earliest form of modern chemistry, and it explores the nature of substances. Physically, alchemy is the process of transmuting base metals—aluminum, copper, lead—into gold by heating the base metals with fire. Throughout the transmutation process, the fire's different flame colors indicate the progression of the change. The pearlescent flame, which holds within it all other colors, is the last before that transmutation is complete. Of course, the alchemists were not successful in their quest, but studying them made me wonder: how could I use the concept of this flame process *internally* to transmute my own beauty?

Internal alchemy leads to an epiphany of personal awakening. Think of it as transmuting the base metal of your thoughts, beliefs, and attitudes into gold. To do this, you have to look at what tools each flame can offer you to dissolve old beliefs, patterns, and impurities and replace them with higher-level thoughts and emotions. Each flame gets you closer to the all-encompassing pearlescent flame—the point at which you can truly "live beautiful."

The Pearlescent Flame: Living Beautiful tells the story of Peregrine, a fictional character who is on a quest to determine her definition of "living beautiful"—or living out the embodiment of what she believes to be true beauty. She does this (often unwittingly) by learning about herself and the world within the matrix of the different alchemical flame processes. Each flame color represents the next phase in her transmutation, bringing about a new experience, a new learning process, and a new understanding about what "living beautiful" means in her life.

True beauty comes from nourishing your mind, your body, and your spirit. It is my life's work to help others reach a place of clarity, understanding, and acceptance in which they can expand their definitions of beauty. So many of us buy into a manufactured idea of beauty, unconsciously giving away our power to define it for ourselves. We accept that if we do not meet society's ideals, we are *not* beautiful. This is nothing short of tragic, especially considering that physical concepts of beauty are ever evolving.

I hope you will not only enjoy Peregrine's journey but—through debriefs and reader questions at the end of each chapter—also learn to incorporate internal alchemy into your own life. There is no greater freedom than embracing your authentic self and giving yourself permission to live beautiful.

—Jessica Puckett
Internal alchemist

CHAPTER 1

Red Flame: Hometown

RED FLAME: *The red flame wants to illuminate the nature of our true being. We use this flame to highlight the root of our authentic self and to master self-expression.*

Peregrine shook her red hair out from its ponytail. Finally. She let her waves cascade over the black lace sleeves of her dress and down the white mink stole. She'd only just discarded the jeans and sweatshirt that had hidden her all week when she heard the familiar *click clack, click clack* down the hall. A slight knock followed.

"Are you ready for our cinematic evening?" Mimi asked.

Peregrine's grandmother was a ruby flame, a career woman with one child in the era of Jackie Kennedy. Timeless in her Chanel suits and pearls, she wore high heels well into her seventies and loved when Peregrine, fourteen and in love with all things beautiful, first clomped, then glided across the master bathroom in them. Mimi couldn't restrain a soft smile when Peregrine reached for the jade sculptures in the formal dining room or admired the Georgia O'Keefe that hung over the fireplace.

All week long, Peregrine slopped around the house she shared with her parents and two younger brothers. She went to school in jeans and a ponytail, did her homework on a plain oak desk pushed against a white wall, and climbed trees with her brothers in the evenings out of boredom. She longed for aesthetics and found she had more to talk about with Mimi than she ever could with her mother or any of the girls at school. She couldn't wait for weekends, when she could unabashedly dress up in Mimi's glamorous vintage pieces and then curl up with her grandmother on the couch for movies and actual *interesting* conversation. Mimi's house was a different world—vibrant and rich—than the one Peregrine inhabited every day.

"What movie are we watching tonight?" Peregrine asked.

Mimi smiled. "How about *Nosferatu?*"

Peregrine nodded eagerly, following Mimi into the living room. They settled onto a large, deep-cushioned couch, cuddling close beneath a cashmere blanket. Mimi pressed play on the remote, and soon Peregrine was losing herself in dark and shadowy images. She often had to squint to make out the hem of a cloak, just before the character leapt onscreen and made Peregrine jump with startled delight.

"You know these movies aren't just about vampires, don't you?" Mimi asked.

Peregrine tore her gaze away from the long-nailed monster on screen. Mimi's eyes were dancing, and she knew her grandmother had more to say. "What are they about?"

"The unknown," Mimi said. "They explore personal boundaries. They tell us there's something mysterious in the world, something we can't see."

Peregrine wasn't entirely sure what Mimi meant, but she nodded and imagined being able to slip away a veil and see into the unknown. What would be revealed? *Just because we can't prove certain things exist doesn't mean they don't*, Peregrine thought. The idea frightened and excited her.

"Even people," Mimi added. "There's more behind them than what you see."

Mimi winked, and Peregrine smiled. She knew her grandmother was talking about her—there was more to Peregrine than she allowed anyone but Mimi to see. She lived in her mind, far away from the petty judgment of others.

The time not spent in the oasis of her grandparents' home was otherwise awkward and stilted. Peregrine's father—a kind, gentle soul—would walk on water for anyone who needed it. He was a giver, a shy middle child Peregrine had connected with more as a little girl than she did now. She remembered sitting in his lap and eating popcorn with him as they watched *Johnny Carson* late at night, eventually falling asleep in his arms. A too-young marriage and a baby a year as he transitioned from boy to man had left him with little time to fulfill his own dreams. It wasn't until now, when Peregrine was a teenager, that he decided to take a risk and earn a bachelors, then masters, degree while working full-time to support the family. As Peregrine grew older and clamored for independence, they drifted apart.

Peregrine's mother, the only child of Mimi and Grandpa, had rebelled against Mimi's urgings for a "big" life, instead marrying young and settling into a predictable suburban routine. This would have been fine if it were truly what Peregrine's mother wanted, but her decisions were transparent: she simply wanted to make all the opposite choices as Mimi. Peregrine sometimes had trouble believing that her mother ever occupied the same space as Mimi, much less came from her body. Peregrine's mother was awkward in every way that Mimi was graceful. Her ill-fitting jeans and unintentionally blunt haircut frustrated Peregrine to almost the same extreme that Mimi's glamour excited her—and it wasn't just about looks. It wasn't about Peregrine feeling embarrassed of her mother's bad wardrobe. It was that her mother was trapped in a state of teenage rebellion, living a life of settlement and not one of dreams.

The tragedy of both Peregrine's parents was that they were incredibly smart, creative people who decided to merge their lives together without having developed their own authentic personalities first. Peregrine was convinced that if only her mother could access the fine qualities she had in her soul, she could exude a different energy, one of passion and beauty. But she didn't. Most people around her didn't, Peregrine was realizing. There had to be more in the world— people who thought differently, looked differently—than what she saw in her southern hometown.

In high school, Peregrine was introverted but had a few friends in her art classes. There was Andrew, her childhood friend and sometimes-boyfriend, as well as Todd, of whom she was especially fond. Todd was mostly quiet, like her, but their exchanges had always been pleasant, and they mutually admired each other's work. Although Peregrine wouldn't say that she and Todd were *close*, she always respected his authenticity. She was envious of his ability to be so true to himself—diving into his art, wearing a suit one day and goth clothes the next—despite the taunts and occasional black eye from classmates who didn't understand.

One day, when shuffling between classes, she saw a gathering of students in the hallway. Never one to engage in gossip, she kept moving. Then she glimpsed familiar blue hair.

"Faggot!"

Peregrine froze, her eyes wide. She watched Todd being beaten, his head repeatedly slammed into a locker. He had been dating Marjorie since their freshman year. Of all the names in the world, this stupid jock was calling Todd a "faggot," just because he dressed differently.

Peregrine's disbelief quickly turned to anger. *This* was why she felt she had to quietly glide across the hallways in school. *This* was why she rarely left the art room. The level of acceptance for anyone not wearing the same stupid Gap sweaters was nonexistent. Not only were students judged physically on their appearance, they were judged personally for any choices that deviated from the "norm."

"I've got a girlfriend, man," Todd protested. "Please. What did I ever do to you?"

"You're in *my* school," replied the jock. "Why should I have to look at your weird clothes? Your punk hair? You want to stand out? Well, here it is."

Peregrine knew she should say something. She should intercede on Todd's behalf. At the same time, she knew it was useless. Nothing would change. She knew Todd felt the same way—they couldn't wait to be out of high school. The ecosystem of tardy bells and conformity would surely not outlast these hallways. When she was free from this place, there would be a place for her in the world, and there would be a place for Todd, too. He was lucky that he was already a senior. She still had another year in this hellhole.

With a brief, sympathetic meeting of Todd's eyes, Peregrine hurried to her next class.

After packing herself into a box five days a week, Peregrine craved her Friday nights at Mimi's house. Like Peregrine, Mimi was a night owl. Instead of staring at the ceiling and listening to Pink Floyd well past her usual weeknight ten p.m. lights-out, Peregrine was free to watch the movies she had loved for years. The idea of being pushed to the limit of one's existence also translated into other media for Peregrine. She devoured Victorian Gothic literature, existential philosophy, and aesthetic literature. Ann Radcliff, Mary Shelley, Oscar Wilde, and Sartre were among the authors stacked on her nightstand.

The search for mental stimulation was only part of the reasoning behind the movies she and Mimi selected. Deep down, both Peregrine and Mimi longed to be as visually pleased as they were intrigued. One of their favorite films to watch together was *Do You Love Me*. Peregrine, growing up in the age of rap videos and MTV's Spring Break, was excited to see a different idea of femininity and personality. Not only did Maureen O'Hara have gorgeous fiery red hair, her character also learned to embrace her femininity without losing her intelligence or spirit.

"Those were the good old days," Mimi said. "Women weren't afraid to be women. They were feminine *and* strong. They dressed as women, and men were actually *gentlemen*."

Peregrine nodded. She soaked up the wit in the characters' exchanges, longing for this reality. She wanted nothing more than to live in a world where she could choose to be brassy, artistic, and beautiful out loud ... after all, this was already her internal reality. Vaguely, she realized she was searching for her beauty in an impossibly bland world; how would she possibly find herself *here*, in this small town outside New Orleans that no one ever seemed to leave?

After the movie, Peregrine went upstairs for a bubble bath in Mimi's oversized tub. When she was younger, she would emerge from the tub and wrap herself in an oversized fluffy towel. Then Mimi would give her a massage with different scented lotions before allowing her to play with a big jewelry box. Peregrine had never tired of sifting through the gold and silver inside. With careful, almost reverent fingers, she layered delicate pendants with bold, chunky necklaces and stretched her neck in the mirror, admiring how each metal or stone caught the light in a different way. She slipped her wrists through a half dozen bracelets and held up earrings that she sensed couldn't be bought at just any jewelry store. Mimi's jewelry was a collection. It was art, carefully curated as she lived her life. To Peregrine, the jewelry implied a story. It was discreet—a whisper, not a shout—of Mimi's journey, of how she'd become the feminist fashionista that she was and what identities she'd explored along the way.

Mimi's perfumes in their beautiful old bottles held a similar fascination for Peregrine. Knowing there was only a finite amount of liquid inside, Peregrine took care not to spray them frivolously, but she often held them up to her nose and breathed deeply the wide variety of their scents. Some of them felt dark and mysterious to her, like something a woman might wear on a clandestine date, while others were floral and fruity, instantly lifting her mood. She wondered about the stories behind the different scents, but she never asked Mimi about them. Something about smell felt personal to Peregrine.

During her junior year of high school, Peregrine was able to turn her eye for beauty into a job. While helping her mother with ceramics, she started making porcelain dolls by order. She rented booths at crafts fairs and found that she was able to bring in between three hundred and five hundred dollars for one doll! This was the catalyst she had been looking for: a way to turn her artistic abilities into cash that would eventually buy her freedom.

She bought her own second-hand car and drove out of town, often and alone. The simplicity of the other girls at school made it impossible for Peregrine to achieve a connection with them. While she would rather check out a new gallery or have coffee twenty minutes away in New Orleans, her "girlfriends" wanted to use her car to cruise around town and spy on their boyfriends: were they *really* at the football game? Did anyone know who drove the Chevy parked in Joe's driveway? It was ridiculous and made any girls' night Peregrine attempted trite and unnecessary.

One morning, at the end of her junior year, Peregrine pulled into the parking lot of her high school a few minutes late. She was exhausted from adorning a special order doll until the wee hours, and she sipped black tea as she hurried to the art room. It was, by all accounts, a typical morning, yet something felt different. Then she realized: those who were usually oblivious to her were watching her walk from her car. The jocks in their Top-Siders and varsity jackets gave her sidelong glances. A wall of preps in Ralph Lauren polo shirts lined the hallway. *What is this?*

Peregrine wondered, almost aloud. She did a quick mental inventory of her morning routine and a quick lookover to make sure she hadn't spilled her tea or gotten glue on her clothes from the dolls she made the night before. *Maybe this is what Todd feels like all the time*, she thought. While she did envy his ability to be true to himself, she knew this strange attention was precisely what she didn't want. This was why she worked so carefully to pack herself away at the start of each school day.

In the art room, the scene was much the same as it was in the hallway. No radio humming along to The Beatles, no oblivious artists buzzing about. In fact, it was silent, and everyone turned as she entered.

"Sorry I'm late," Peregrine said. It was out of character for her to say anything announcing her entrance, but the energy in the room begged to be broken by something.

Her teacher made way to the door. Her eyes were red-rimmed, and her voice broke as she began, "Peregrine, it's Todd."

"Todd? What about him?"

"He's ... He ... He's no longer with us." Her teacher burst into tears. The sobs came so easily, so freely.

"What?"

"He, well, he chose to take his own life."

Peregrine's vision blurred. Todd? *Todd*? They had to be wrong. Todd wouldn't do that. How could someone so un-afraid of himself be so afraid of the world that he chose to leave it? She had a million questions, for which there would never be answers, because they weren't wrong; Todd had shot himself the night before.

She walked out of the classroom, climbed into her car, and drove straight back home. Since no one was there, she could be alone for a while. She thought of calling Mimi, but she didn't really want to hear what Mimi thought about this. She was beyond consolation, beyond tears, beyond reason. After lying in her bed all afternoon, Peregrine realized that she needed to get out of the house before her mother returned.

In the car—the car she thought brought her so much freedom—she realized how restricted she still was. She moved with the traffic. Stop. Go. Turn. Yield. She wasn't actually paying attention to the road. She was just going through the motions to get to her destination. Then it hit her: this was all she'd been doing. For almost eighteen years. *She stops, she goes. She wears jeans and sweaters, and she slides on shoes. She climbs trees with her brothers. She conjugates Latin verbs for a test.* There was no more Peregrine in any action of any given day then there was in her driving right now. She was allowing herself to become one of them—consciously choosing to be something other than herself.

Suddenly, she drove with awareness. She saw the trees lining the highway. She listened to "Dark Side of the Moon" on her car stereo. Finally, she pulled into the closest parking spot by her favorite boutique. She decided that her life deserved to be lived.

In the store, which she had frequented with dreams but never a wallet, she found everything she liked. She tried on vintage Chanel dresses and four-inch heels. She found gorgeous art deco earrings that were almost as big as her fist. She took these things, and more, with abandon to the register, pulling out the wad of cash that she'd been saving to make her grand escape. This was it; this was her choice to start living out loud.

Once she got home, she admired her reflection in the full-length mirror she'd gotten for Christmas. In the past, she'd reserved her beautiful things—many handed down from Mimi—for weekend life while she poured over Nietzsche, sipping espresso. But what did it matter if people commented on her clothes? What could anyone say that would truly hurt her? She was tired of containing her spirit. Besides, it was the people who were living their lives for society who had killed Todd. She couldn't be one of those people, not even just in public. She had to do this, for Todd, for herself, and for everyone else who lived in their minds. Peregrine may not be "good enough" according to her high school social norms, but she quit caring and decided she would live her life authentically.

"I am who I am," she whispered to her reflection in the mirror, "and no one else has to understand."

Debrief

CALCINATION: THE RED FLAME

Most of us develop a belief system about ourselves that is largely defined by society—we're too much of this or two little of that, imperfect and unworthy. Those negative thoughts often take over our subconscious mind, where the connection with our true self lies. In the process of internal alchemy, we have reached the first phase of transmutation: calcination, the red flame. The red flame is the first awakening to your true inner beauty. We are looking at what makes up our authentic selves. How do we live that out?

Look at yourself. Do you hide your authentic self? ꙮ Do you follow the norm to fit in? ꙮ What are the self-imposed beliefs and limitations that are working in your life? ꙮ What or who helped form these beliefs? ꙮ Why do you feel that you can't be your authentic self? ꙮ Do your actions reflect true *choice*? ꙮ Do you own your life and your beauty? Here is your first chance to *choose* to live authentically.

Be the Phoenix. Burn down your old beliefs and rise from the ashes anew.

CHAPTER 2

Orange Flame: Paris

ORANGE FLAME: *The deep orange glow of this flame illuminates the space between magic and science. This is where closely-linked sexuality and creativity are born. This flame will manifest beauty through the healthy balance of desire, passion, creativity, and sexuality.*

Once Peregrine realized the art of self-expression, the universe became more open to her. She no longer tried to hide who she was or to be something she was not. She was thankful to Todd for his example and only wished that he could see the authenticity he sparked in her.

Peregrine spent her senior year in the art room. She managed to arrange her classes so that they were mostly art electives, allowing her to spend days in the darkroom or painting her porcelain dolls. Business was booming; she made enough money to support her fashion habit and restart a getaway fund. The only restrictions placed on her now were those of her hometown, and she knew she would outgrow those. That knowledge gave her a refreshing sense of freedom.

Peregrine's mother was not terribly impressed with her newfound sense of independence. She argued that Peregrine was nothing more than a second-rate Mimi—that Peregrine was projecting herself as a starlet when, in reality, she was just a typical high school kid. Her mother never hesitated to remind Peregrine of how she and her father strove to provide her with a childhood free of pressure to be anything extraordinary. The comments were truly ironic. Now that Peregrine had begun the escape from her incorrectly informed ego, her mother was angry that Peregrine was everything she had rebelled against. Now she was judging Peregrine with the same furiousness that she'd felt when judged by Mimi as a girl. Peregrine wanted out.

No sooner had she graduated than she moved into her own one-bedroom apartment in the French Quarter. It was a divided 1920s house with high ceilings, tall windows, and hardwood floors. French doors opened to a little balcony that overlooked the neighborhood coffee house and offered a glimpse of the trendy new restaurants down the street. Some of the city's grittier residences were just a few blocks over. Peregrine felt that moving into the city's urban center was one more act of breaking free.

A minimalist at heart, Peregrine carefully arranged her antique marble-topped table; a long, low sofa reupholstered with green velvet and buttons down the back; and the antique Asian table she used as a coffee table—all gifts from Mimi or things the two had picked out while antiquing together. She had a little stand for the TV and an armoire-style desk for her computer, and the dining room was just large enough for her antique Duncan Phyfe table as long as she folded down one leaf and pushed it against the wall. Her dishes fit into the apartment's built-in hutches, and the kitchen had just enough space for her pots and pans and what canned and boxed food she cared to keep on the shelf.

The bedroom was large enough only for a simple, full-size iron bed, with her dresser tucked into a closet at the end of the room. One huge, ornate-framed mirror bounced the light and visually enlarged the space. With a few pieces of photography and art on the walls, her decorating job was finished. Peregrine didn't believe in knick-knacks. A sparse design scheme with a few good pieces of furniture refreshed her and put her heart at ease.

As she rounded out her freshman year of college, Peregrine couldn't wait one minute longer to explore the world. At nineteen, she wanted to discover who she was when her family and friends weren't around to label her with familiar descriptors. Peregrine held a dream in her pocket: this was the summer she would go to Paris. She had enough in her getaway fund to leave when she wanted to and stay for ten days. She felt no compunction to tell anyone where she was going; after all, she only spoke with her parents every couple of weeks. In a new place, she wouldn't even have to give people her real name if she didn't want to. The idea made her giddy.

Her flight was still weeks away when Peregrine started packing her most stylish dresses and shoes. She lovingly stroked her silk cloche with the peacock feathers and remembered what the popular girls in high school had said the first time she wore it to class: "Just who do you think you are, Peregrine?" The words had been meant to make her feel badly about herself, but the question was central to Peregrine's thoughts of the moment: who *was* she, really?

Immediately following her chemistry final, Peregrine called a cab to take her to the airport. She had a window seat on the plane, just as she'd requested. She would soon arrive in New York and later depart for Paris. In the next twenty-four hours, she could toy with creating a whole new identity.

As the plane's nose stretched toward the sky, Peregrine thought of Mimi—she would be the only one able to understand Peregrine's need to leave and to explore herself. And Paris! How often had Peregrine fantasized about Paris as she played with Mimi's classic perfumes and jewelry or during the many nights they'd spent curled in front of black and white movies set in Paris? Peregrine gazed at the shadows the clouds cast on the flat land below. The shadows were almost spooky. Mimi and Grandpa would appreciate that, she thought. They loved to create a mysterious environment with their old gothic movies and ghost stories, and they often waited in doorways to jump out and scare Peregrine and her brothers. They loved to play with the idea of the supernatural but also had a deep religious faith. Through them, Peregrine had learned that the unknown, the undefined, was a grand place to explore the mysteries of life. She was heading for that unknown.

Twelve hours later, as her cab brought her from the de Gaulle airport to her hotel in the Sixth Arrondissement, Peregrine's smile started to hurt her cheeks. She peered through the windows at centuries-old buildings that pedestrians passed without notice. The buildings were older than anything she had ever seen in the States. She couldn't believe she was here.

She paid the cab driver and tipped him with the French banknotes she'd special-ordered back home, having studied the exchange rate along with her tour guides. She was glad she'd packed relatively lightly as she carried her suitcases up five flights of stairs at her hotel.

In her room, Peregrine dropped her luggage and pulled back the drapes from the window. The almost-unreal city-scape across the Seine stretched before her, and Peregrine's view swam with tears. There was so much opportunity and possibility in the world, and here it was, lying at her feet. Here, in Paris, were people Peregrine would never have known existed had she not boarded that plane. Of course, the same was true even back home; how many amazing people would she be oblivious to in her life? The thought jolted Peregrine from her reverie. Why was she just *thinking* about this? She was in Paris! She was free to make her own reality.

Despite jet lag, Peregrine quickly unpacked and hung her dresses in the antique chifforobe. She draped a cream-colored silk dress with violet flowers on a hanger and hung it from the shower curtain rod. Stepping out of her travel-ing clothes and into the claw-foot iron tub, she took a hot shower to perk up and simultaneously steam the wrinkles from her dress. A few minutes later, wearing the refreshed dress, a cute pair of heels that she'd broken in back home, and her favorite silk cloche with the peacock feathers, she admired herself in the hotel mirror. Her long, wavy ginger hair, blue eyes, and peaches-and-cream complexion made her look young and energetic. She grabbed her purse with its new red arrondissement book—and the French *Vogue* she'd bought at the airport—and set off for her first mini-adventure.

Down the Boulevard Saint Germain, she found a classic-looking café that appeared to cater to locals as well as tourists.

"*Bonjour*," Peregrine greeted the *maître d'*.

The thin, dark-haired man smiled. "*Bonjour. Comment allez-vous?*"

How are you was one of the few French phrases Peregrine knew. She smiled back. "*Bien, merci.*"

Following the *maître d'*, she selected a seat along the sidewalk with the best view and ordered herself a glass of champagne. What bliss, for a nineteen-year-old to drink champagne in the middle of the day in a gorgeous café on the Left Bank!

Sitting alongside the wrought-iron fence that separated the café patrons from the pedestrians, Peregrine studied the people at surrounding tables as unobtrusively as possible. Mostly, they seemed to be native Parisians and Europeans. Everyone, no matter how animated, was speaking in genteel tones, oozing style and sophistication regardless of what they were wearing. They wore clothes as if they believed their outfits were the best things they could possibly pull from their closets. Across the aisle from Peregrine, one woman's hair was pulled up messily with a scarf. She hardly wore any makeup besides some light lipstick, but her pearls and the natural light shining out of her eyes made her look amazingly chic and poised.

Sipping her champagne and sighing with contentment, Peregrine opened her satchel and pulled out her travel book of Parisian arrondissements, or neighborhoods, to plan the next day's shopping trip. She looked up to lift the glass of champagne to her lips and noticed a striking man about twenty feet ahead of her. He wasn't walking toward *her*, in particular, but down the sidewalk next to the iron fence at her shoulder. He was medium height, about five feet eight inches, with black hair that swooped over one eye to his cheekbone, piercing light blue eyes, and a long straight nose. *Dang*, Peregrine thought. She'd only had one glass of champagne, but she knew that it and this man approaching were a dangerous combination! In that moment, she wanted nothing more than stop the man and tell him exactly what she was thinking. Oh, the choices to make in a split-second!

Her heart pounded with familiar introversion as the man reached her table. This was it. Here, now, she would let go of who she had been back home and embrace who she could be in Paris.

"Excuse me," Peregrine said.

He stopped. "Yes?"

"You have the prettiest eyes I think I have ever seen on a man," she told him, her gaze direct. "Would you please sit down with me for a cup of coffee or glass of champagne?"

He gave her a small but curious smile, and she continued. "Because I can't stand for those eyes to go away until I can look at them a little longer." She felt her cheeks flush, not quite believing she'd said the words aloud, but she didn't break eye contact.

For a moment, he just stood there. Then he appeared to make a decision. "My name is Alexandre. What is yours?"

Two minutes later, he was seated across the table from her. Each held a full glass of champagne, toasting. The power of the moment, the power of choice, the fact that she had effectively picked up this handsome Frenchman, empowered and excited Peregrine.

Alexandre asked why she had visited Paris, where she was from, and how long she was staying. "Who let loose such a beautiful woman, alone, in Paris—the most romantic city in the world?"

"Isn't it unfair to cage a tiger?" she asked playfully.

He smiled. "Are you a tiger?"

"It depends whom you ask on what day." Peregrine was flushed and heady. Where was she *getting* this? She almost giggled at their banter.

Alexandre laughed and leaned forward. "If you don't mind, how old are you, Peregrine?"

Hesitating only slightly, she said, "I'm twenty-three." She sat back in her chair, gave him her best poker face, and willed herself not to blush. Peregrine gauged Alexandre's age at about thirty-two, so even with her little white lie, he still had experience on his side.

He gazed at her for a moment. Seemingly satisfied, he reached out to tuck her hair behind her ear. Softly, he ran a fingertip down her jaw. "I should get back to my office, but may I take you out to dinner tomorrow night?"

She almost leapt across the table to say yes but allowed a coolness to wash over her and keep her in her seat. After getting the name of her hotel and settling on a time to pick her up, Alexandre rose, kissed her hand, and was gone.

Oh my god, Peregrine thought, grinning as she sipped her

champagne. She was no virgin, but she'd never pursued a man before or been so immediately intimate with a stranger. The openness was blissfully freeing, an intensified version of the way she used to feel when she pulled her hair from its boring daily ponytail. And this was just the first day!

Feeling a little tipsy from the champagne and the interaction with the handsome Alexandre, Peregrine ordered an espresso and then wandered to another cafe for an early dinner of duck confit. She spent the next few hours exploring the small boutiques that lined the Rue de Vaugirard before ending up at a bar near her hotel. There, she was invited to join a table full of young travelers from Australia, Germany, and South America. She was still giddy, enjoying her first night in the city, but feeling the effects of the time zone shift. She stayed out until one a.m. and then made it back to her room to sleep quite soundly. Her dreams that night were full of possibilities.

. . .

In the morning, Peregrine visited the Eiffel Tower and then went shopping on the Avenue des Champs-Elysées. With only minute hesitation, she strode into Yves Saint Laurent as if she owned it. She knew that nothing in the store was under a thousand dollars, and she willed herself not to look at price tags as she admired purses and shoes. She held up a pair of bronze strappy sandals with a dangerously thin stiletto heel and smiled at the saleslady.

"May I try these in a thirty-nine?" she asked.

The sandals looked even better on her feet than in her hand, and she admired them in the mirror for a full five minutes. She pictured herself saying, "I'll take them. Have them delivered to my suite!" But she didn't have to own the shoes to enjoy the pleasure of imagining possibilities.

Around the corner, she found a smaller, slightly less-pricy store with a drop-dead gorgeous red dress in the window. Entering, she pointed at the dress and asked, "Do you have this in a size . . ." She converted the U.S. size four to French sizing. ". . . thirty-six?"

The shopkeeper, a chic woman about Peregrine's mother's age with glossy, long brunette hair pulled up into a loose twist, smiled broadly and pulled the dress from the mannequin. "This is our last copy of this dress. My dear, with your red hair, you'll be making quite a statement!"

"Isn't that the point?" Peregrine laughed. "For a redhead to be in a red dress, there is some serious business to be done!"

The shopkeeper smiled and ushered Peregrine into a tiny dressing room. "My name is Francoise. Do you have a special occasion in mind for this gown?"

"I have a date tonight with a man I met yesterday!" Peregrine shared, slipping off her shoes and dress. Francoise averted her eyes and held out the dress, waiting to raise the zipper. The dress was ruby-colored silk with a deep vee neckline and a plunging back. One strap wrapped over Peregrine's shoulder to hold the bodice in place. The vision in the mirror nearly took Peregrine's breath away.

With a knowing smile, Francoise said, "I'm sure this man won't be able to tear his eyes—or his hands—off you."

Peregrine grinned with that exact hope in mind. "I'll take it."

Within a few moments, she'd paid for the dress and grabbed a cab back to her hotel. She took her time showering and doing her hair and makeup, and when she was dressed, she gazed at herself in the mirror with surprise. She felt light-years away from the girl who once dressed to blend in with her high school classmates. She looked like a woman. A real woman—one who knew herself exactly. Tonight she was going to live in that knowing.

Right on time, the hotel phone buzzed to let her know that Alexandre was in the lobby. His eyes widened appreciatively as Peregrine walked downstairs, and he rose immediately from his seat and kissed her hand. He gave her his arm and led her to his car on the street. He made a point to drive past the Moulin Rouge, and soon they pulled up in front of a gorgeous restaurant in Montmartre.

Inside, the *maître d'* led them past a series of dimly lit, velvet-upholstered booths towards a similar cozy enclave in the back of the room. Peregrine slipped into the booth, scooting carefully but not without poise in her tight dress. The waiter left them with menus, and she handed hers to Alexandre. She couldn't have cared less what they ate.

"I trust you to order for us both," she said.

Alexandre and the waiter exchanged French too fast for her to follow, and soon, plate after plate of delectable dishes were brought to the table.

He showed her how to grasp the beautiful, coiled snail shells with the special tool and pluck out the oily, garlic-laden meat with a tiny fork. He offered it to her, and Peregrine delicately took it into her mouth.

"Oh," she said, surprised by how much she liked it.

Alexandre watched with amusement. "Now sip champagne." He tilted the fluted glass toward her. Then, as

Peregrine reveled in the delicious flavor, he leaned in to kiss her. His lips were both soft and firm. They carried a sense of gentle power. "This is the proper way to eat snails," he murmured. "A snail, a sip, and a kiss."

After that, they shared each dish and spent as much time drinking champagne and kissing as they did eating their meal.

"I seem to have run into a streak of luck, being able to introduce you to the delights of Paris on your first visit to France," Alexandre said.

Peregrine gazed into his eyes. "Seems like I'm the lucky one to be on the receiving end of your delights." Before she lost her nerve, she added, "And I'm looking forward to receiving many more." She smiled and took another sip of champagne.

Peregrine was buzzing with energy as she played with her sexuality over dinner. It was a game, a challenge, and she had never felt so free. She also couldn't help appreciating how freely Alexandre gave of himself and inspired her to do the same. He was intimate but not groping; the quiet confidence of his hands and lips was so different from anyone she'd dated back home. As they continued to drink champagne and feed each other tidbits from the plates, savoring flavors and sensations––not to mention kisses and caresses––she thought, *There's an art to this: giving and accepting.* Then she thought, *I want to go home with him—and I don't even remember his last name!* A part of her recognized that she was taking chances, but in the moment, she could only revel in her own freedom and power and this newfound sexual expression. This risk was one she felt was worth taking.

After dinner, they walked arm in arm back to his car. The evening air was warm against Peregrine's skin, and the lighted Parisian nightscape cast a warm romantic glow between them.

"Are you ready to return to your hotel?" Alexandre asked.

"No. I want to go back to *your* hotel."

He chuckled. "I don't have a hotel. I live here, remember?"

"Well, you have a room, don't you? An apartment or something?"

Alexandre's full lips curved into a delicious smile as he opened her car door. "Of course I do."

Peregrine ran the tips of her fingers over his knuckles as he drove them farther west into a quieter, more residential part of the city. Arriving in his apartment—chic and minimalist—Alexandre led Peregrine to a balcony off his living room. He gestured toward a small café table as he assembled a tray with two glasses and a bottle of Cognac. Before they finished even one small glass, they were in each other's arms.

For the next few hours, every part of Peregrine was open and confident, welcoming his touch and his gaze. He was both gentle and passionate, exploring Peregrine's body in a way that inspired her to return the intimacy. "You are so beautiful," he said, his fingertips stroking the length of her body. The windows were open, and the sounds of the city—the soft whir of traffic, footsteps down the street—were a backdrop to the rustling of sheets and the rise and fall of their breath. A couple giggled as they passed Alexandre's building, as though they were on their way to their own rendezvous. Every now and then, a whisper of a breeze cooled the perspiration on Peregrine's skin and lifted the scent of Alexandre's cologne. It was woodsy, earthy, with the subtle undercurrent of his natural musk. As they kissed, she tasted cognac on his tongue. His skin under her lips was warm, and though the room was dim, the lights of the city illuminated the desire in his blue eyes. The evening passed as though she were in a trance, at once utterly alive and yet completely relaxed. She had never experienced sexual freedom like this.

In the morning, she woke to the smell of fresh coffee: he'd awakened before her to make her a bonne femme omelet and coffee and served it on the balcony where they could enjoy the view of the city by the morning light. He drove her back to her hotel around eleven.

"I have to leave the city for a week on business," he said, bringing the car to a stop. "I'd love to see you again when I return." He smiled, touching her face with his gentle hands.

"I'd love to." Peregrine leaned over to kiss him. As she slipped from the car, she simultaneously believed that he would call and didn't care if he did. She understood that this would be a short-lived affair—and she was okay with that. She had gotten everything she needed at this time from the experience.

Upstairs in the bath, Peregrine reveled in memories of last night and marveled at herself. That man—that *beautiful* man—believed she was sexy because she had *allowed* herself to *be* sexy. She had dripped with sensuality, as if no one could compare to her. The marvelous thing, she realized now, was that she believed it, too—and it had been inside her all along. She didn't have to go halfway around the world to access this power; she could conjure it up anytime. And she owed it to herself. The flame of change was glowing inside of her, sparking a revolution of creativity and inspiration through the beauty of sensuality. The world—*her* world—was changing; it was more alive and full of exciting possibilities.

Peregrine rose from the warm water and wrapped herself in a towel. She wiped steam from the mirror and looked at her sparkling, intensely blue eyes. What other identities, she wondered, were inside her, waiting to be unfurled? She felt herself emerging as if from a cocoon and enjoyed the vision of herself stretching open her wings at last. What else was waiting to be discovered?

Today, she decided, she'd begin exploring the perfumeries of the city. After experiencing last night's selected hedonism—a dress that felt like heaven caressing her skin, dinner consisting of a symphony of flavors, champagne that danced on her palate, and a phenomenal exploration of her sexuality with Alexandre—it was time to indulge her sense of smell.

In each *parfumerie*, she expanded the knowledge that had begun early in her life with Mimi's tray of perfumes on top of her dressing table. When she was a little girl, before realizing how precious those scents were, Peregrine had squeezed the bulbs on Mimi's old atomizers to spray the perfumes on her wrists, clothes, and hair. To her, the bottles were amazing pieces of sculpture filled with magical elixirs that transported her thoughts and emotions. For Peregrine, all of life's mysteries could conceivably be wrapped up in the olfactory system; what a good perfume could unlock in the mind held a deep fascination for her.

At the first parfumerie, the tour guide explained, "Perfume is like a musical symphony, with base notes, middle notes, top notes, and the space between each of those notes. As in music, the silence between the notes is just as important as the notes themselves."

Peregrine smiled, imagining the mist of perfume the guide sprayed as a stream of musical notes only she could hear.

"Perfumes smell differently with time, as each note diffuses at different rates," the parfumerie guide explained. The group trailed behind him. "It's what we call the 'dry down effect.' In addition, any given perfume combines with a woman's varied body chemistry to smell unique on each woman and to smell different on a single woman at different times of the month."

In the parfumerie's equivalent of a winery tasting room, Peregrine learned how to identify the basic components of each layer and began to play with layering scents that pleased her into her own custom perfume. She discovered that her preferences were what perfumers called Orientals: deep amber scents reminiscent of musks, woods, vanillas, tobaccos, leathers. Florals, for Peregrine, felt ephemeral—only beautiful for a second before they disintegrated. They almost made her feel uneasy; some smelled so sweet it was putrid, like rotting flesh.

"Because flowers are always on the verge of death, every single second has an intense vulnerability," the guide said. "In contrast, woody scents create a feeling of stability, endurance, and wisdom. Think of a tree. There are trees that are thousands of years old on this earth, and they are the givers and sustainers of life. Meanwhile, grassy notes come forth from a very hard earth with a fresh vivacity and energy. It is as if they are saying, 'You can cut me down and cut me down, and I will come back again and again, always with a fresh outlook.' Every scent category has its own energetic properties. Each has a story to tell."

Peregrine had intuited so much about the power of perfumes, and this trip was providing her the language to support that. As she listened to the guide put words to her unspoken feelings, she knew that she wanted a place in this beautifully scented world. She wanted to learn more about perfumes. She had stories that she wanted to tell.

The tour guide continued. "Perfume conjures up emotions that go so far beyond the fact of the scent. It's your internal alchemy—how you create something in yourself to empower you in that moment. Perfumes can infuse you with all different types of emotions. If you want to feel fresh and clean, wear citrus. That is why citrus scents are good for the summer time—because you perspire, and they make you feel as if you have cleansed yourself." The tour group grinned and nodded. "Lemon, grapefruit, lime—they are refreshing and cleansing. That is why so many household cleaners use those scents."

Going from one small parfumerie to the next, Peregrine decided it was time to step up her game and visit the granddaddy of them all: Guerlain, one of the oldest parfumeries in the world.

The scene reminded her again of the age difference between Europe and America and each continent's varied architectural styles: the surroundings here were art nouveau, glass and mirrors, gold and polished brass. Just walking through the doors felt decadent and transporting. Knowing that the classic parfumerie had all its secrets locked up, Peregrine wasn't sure whether the tour was showing the *actual* rooms where perfumes were concocted or if it was more of a stage show; in either case, the experience was palpably different than any other.

Here, she learned more of the history of perfume—that remnants of perfumes had been found in archeological digs from ancient times, and that in the seventeenth century, only wealthy people used perfumes because the oils were so expensive. When the tour guide explained that many perfumes were created to mask body odors from infrequent bathing, Peregrine grinned. She thought of hippies in the 1960s who used patchouli for much the same reason. It was a shame a lot of people no longer liked the smell, Peregrine thought. According to the tour guide, it was one of the amazing building blocks of perfumery.

"Creating perfume isn't just about dreaming up a scent," the tour guide continued. "It requires precise skill. A perfumer must be able to fixate the formulation so the different notes hold their places, rather than collapse, and diffuse from the skin into the air in a certain pattern. The perfumer must balance a desire for scents to diffuse at different rates against keeping the perfume in a bottle for long periods of time."

In between delivering an education on perfume, the guide wove stories of secret passageways and giant vaults containing Guerlain's recipes. The guide also revealed the perfumer's story behind each scent. Peregrine was enchanted by what felt like a space between magic and science, the perfect place for exploration and creation. She thought of perfumes—all the richness and depth held within—and was transported back to watching those Gothic movies with Mimi. Her grandmother was right. There was magic in the stories and science of the unknown. There was much more to the world than the eye could see.

In Guerlain's gift shop, tourists could purchase anything from its impressive line of perfumes, and they could create their own blend. With the assistance of a *parfumeur* who looked to be her grandfather's age, Peregrine created a scent with woody notes that felt sexy and grounded. This was her Paris scent. She hoped it would transport her back to her discoveries here whenever she wore it.

As she created her perfume, everything the tour guides had explained about scents evoking memories became obvious to her. This was why so many memories of Mimi flashed as she walked past a display of Shalimar and why she felt such a strong sense of love and security whenever she caught a whiff of that perfume. It was not a case of *seeing* beauty but *feeling* it because of a passing scent. She sensed that this was an important understanding—that a scent could evoke an actual *feeling*. When there are feelings, there can be actions.

On her way back to the hotel, Peregrine added one more experience to her day full of olfactory adventures: she stopped into a cigar lounge and asked the barman for his suggestion for a mild, beautiful taste. Following it, she ordered a cigarillo and cognac. The taste and scent of the smoke differed greatly from what she'd smelled from corporate cigars and cigarettes back home. Leaning back in a rich leather chair, Peregrine reflected on her new self-discoveries in Paris: sensuality, passion, creativity, assertiveness, and openness. She knew she had to live out her findings in her everyday life. Peregrine had flown halfway across the world to experience new horizons, but she realized now that it wasn't the geography that made her feel like a different person; it was her choice to shift her attitude and create her own possibilities. It only took a different perspective— a commitment to open, thoughtful explorations—for the world to become new and fresh. It made the prospect of returning home more bearable. The possibility of what life could be extended so far beyond what she'd already lived. The choices were hers to make.

Debrief

DISSOLUTION: ORANGE FLAME

There is an art to giving and receiving pleasure, allowing and rejecting beauty, manifesting passion and creativity, and experiencing it all in a healthy way. This delicate balance is the hallmark of the orange flame. In the orange flame, we come into the realization of the male and female energies that live within us: the soft feminine energies of passion, emotion, sensuality, beauty, and creativity and the male energies of sexuality, desire, initiation, and assertiveness to actualize all those things feminine. The blending of these two forces, like a fine perfume, creates that balance.

We are taught many things about passion and sexuality throughout our lives. Some of us are brought up in rigid belief structures that frame these qualities as taboo. Others are not taught healthy boundaries and experience sexuality without the psychological balance it requires. The pendulum can swing to an unhealthy place either way. The orange flame is the phase of dissolution in the alchemical flame process. Here we have the opportunity to dissolve and break free from mental conditioning and redefine these boundaries for ourselves—to create beauty.

What blocks your sexuality? ∽ Do you think your sexuality is bad, evil, or unhealthy? ∽ Describe how you define beauty and creativity within sexuality. ∽ Is your self-worth and self-esteem tied only to your definition of sexuality? ∽ What is passion to you? What about vitality? Define these words in your terms. ∽ Do you think they are a source of power? ∽ Where and how do you cultivate it? ∽ How is your creativity tied to your passions?

CHAPTER 3

Yellow Flame: New Orleans

YELLOW FLAME: *When the yellow flame burns bright, we are powerful in our own right. This flame is used to clear away insecurities, abuse of power, resentments, and the limitations that come with not seeing our true potential.*

Back home, the summer's humidity enveloped Peregrine in a way that made her weeks in Paris feel like a distant dream. She had been convinced she would never forget what she'd learned about herself and about life, and yet, back in surroundings she'd always known with people who knew her as she'd always been, it was too easy to slide back into her introverted ways. The confident Peregrine of Paris, who was able to attract and seduce a handsome stranger off the street, already felt less accessible.

With two months to kill before sophomore year began, she was working a summer job in Mimi's accounting firm. She spent the hot, muggy days doing general bookkeeping for Mimi's business clients, as well as assisting with basic tax work. It wasn't long before Andrew, her on-and-off boyfriend, saw her car parked outside Mimi's office and left a note under the windshield wiper. "There's a party Saturday night down by the river," he wrote. "You should go. I've missed you."

She and Andrew had been friends since third grade, and he'd spent almost enough time at her house to be thought of as family. Andrew's own family was complicated. His older brother Richard was the star, and even though Andrew would do anything his mother asked of him, he was never good enough in her eyes. Peregrine couldn't understand how he'd abide by that dynamic, but she and her family had taken him under their wings.

As much as Peregrine didn't want to slip into old habits, she had a soft spot for Andrew. At six feet tall, with sandy blond hair, big green eyes, and olive skin, he was the perfect image of a California surfer boy who'd gotten lost in southern America. He was less than driven, but he had a good heart. Peregrine folded the note and slipped it into her purse. Why not? A party could be a decent distraction.

That Saturday, she parked her car with the rest of the beaters and occasional hot rods alongside the county road. She picked her way down a dusty path toward party lights and music in the shelter house down by the river. Andrew must have been watching for her, because before she even got to the edge of the group clustered around a cold keg, he was walking toward her.

"I got in line early for you," he called with a grin, a red Dixie cup in each hand.

Peregrine laughed. "More like I got here at the right time." She accepted the cup and gave him a warm hug.

"You smell good," Andrew said as they pulled away. He

touched her wavy hair. "That's a different perfume you're wearing."

"I made it myself." Peregrine couldn't restrain the pride in her voice. "It's called Pernelle."

"Pernelle?"

"She was the wife of Nicolas Flamel, this famous alchemist in the fifteenth century."

Andrew looked at her blankly.

"I had to learn about the history of chemistry this year," Peregrine explained. "She was quite the interesting character for me."

"Right. So you're a perfume maker now?"

"Well, not quite yet. But maybe one day."

Andrew took her hand. "That's what I love about you. You never do the things everyone else is doing." Before Peregrine could respond or withdraw her hand, he said, "C'mon. Let's walk around."

The crowd looked the same as always: the former jocks loitered near the keg. The ones who hadn't gone on to college looked a bit worn already, and the ones who had didn't seem changed much from the effort; they wore Ralph Lauren polos and boat shoes, chins tilted cockily. The former cheerleaders eyed the group at the keg and watched like vultures for fresh meat arriving from the road. Peregrine steered clear of them, and Andrew remained tethered to her side.

"So," he said. "Typical Peregrine—I heard you didn't tell anyone you went to Paris until after you were back."

She laughed. "No one needed to know."

"Did your parents flip when they found out?"

"Maybe my mom, a little. Mimi just wanted to know why I didn't take her with me. But honestly, no one was really surprised."

Andrew laughed. "So why did you go?"

"Why do you think? I needed to get *out*. I get so tired of seeing the same people, doing the same things, day after day. I wanted to experience something new."

"And did you?"

A secret smile curled Peregrine's lips as she remembered the powerful feelings of beauty she'd cultivated through her sensuality and experienced with Alexandre. Even now, holding a condensation-slippery plastic cup slippery with that was so different from a champagne flute, she felt those feelings stirring inside her. "Paris was beautiful," she said finally. "You should go sometime."

"You know me. I'm comfortable right where I am. This right here—" Andrew gestured expansively, nearly spilling his beer. "This right here is all I need."

She shrugged. If Andrew was happy here, good for him. But she couldn't imagine leading a life she truly desired in this town.

A few minutes later, outside the house, Andrew slipped a flask from a deep pocket and tipped a generous shot of vodka into a Sprite he'd pulled from a cooler.

"Some things never change," she said, thinking of the times they'd done this in the high school parking lot during lunch. They'd pop sticks of gum into their mouths afterwards and head to the art studio, trying not to giggle themselves away.

"Oh, you know it!" He laughed. Then, unexpectedly, his

eyes misted. "You know, though, some things never *should* change."

Here we go, she thought. She took another gulp and leaned against the side of the house, fanning herself with a Bud Light coaster she'd picked up inside. "Change is a good thing. It means we're growing."

"You know what I mean," Andrew said. "We're meant to be together. Deep down, I think you know that. I'll just wait around until you see it, too. I've got time."

. . .

Within a couple of weeks, almost by force, Peregrine had fallen into old habits with Andrew. She had tried to stay distant, but he didn't get the hint, calling and showing up at her house. He needed her, and she didn't want to hurt him. It was co-dependent, Peregrine knew, but she couldn't seem to cut ties. They saw each other every afternoon after she got out of work at Mimi's, and the dynamic between them was the same as it had always been. There was no dynamism, no spark—just familiar comfort. That may have been enough for him, but Peregrine wanted more. However, the more time she spent with him, the further she got from being able to tell him about the deficiencies she felt and the more she knew she needed to.

Andrew's hobby was restoring antique cars. With the care and precision of a surgeon, he stripped them down, restored, and then sold them; he was quite talented in this regard, and Peregrine often watched him work. He moved around his garage with ease, whistling as he reached for the right tools without even looking, green eyes still absorbed in his task. This was the only place he had real confidence, and she so wished it extended outside the small domain.

"You know," she said one afternoon, "you should open your own restoration shop."

Andrew was half buried under the hood of a yellow Porsche. An old Stone Temple Pilots CD played on his stereo. He squinted as he looked up at her. "That'd be nice, but I'm not a businessman. And I don't have the money."

"Well, you can *find* the money," she said. "That's what loans are for. Besides, you do this all the time anyway, and you're already making money. Why not just take it to the next level? I think it'd be good for you."

Andrew wiped his hands on his shorts before taking one of hers. "How about if it's good for *us*?"

Peregrine shook her head. "Maybe one day. For now, let's just focus on you. Is it something you'd want to do?"

"Well . . . yeah. I mean, it beats working for someone else, right? I need to talk to Mom about it, though."

Peregrine fought a roll of her eyes. When would he stop asking for his mother's approval—for her permission to live his life? But this was a step in the right direction. At least he would consider the thought, and she promised to help him raise funds to open the shop if he decided to do it—which, a week later, he did.

As Peregrine should have expected, she was the one who did all the business planning, with little enthusiasm from him. After some time, Andrew called her at home. "Look, I'm tired of talking about the business. I need a break," he said. "A bunch of people are going canoeing this weekend. Want to go?"

Not really paying attention to the phone call, Peregrine marked her page in *The Alchemist*—a necessary reprieve from the spreadsheets she'd been poring over for Andrew's business plan. The last lines she read lingered in her mind: *The alchemists spent years in their laboratories, observing the fire that purified the metals. They spent so much time close to the fire that gradually they gave up the vanities of the world. They discovered that the purification of the metals had led to a purification of themselves.*

"Peregrine?"

"Yeah, sorry. Canoeing. I don't know, Andrew. I'm not really in the mood."

"C'mon, it'll be fun," he said. "The weather will be perfect, we'll do the rapids . . . I'll pick you up Saturday at noon, okay?"

She sighed. She wished she could say no and stick to it, but just imagining the swift change in his voice from hopeful to hurt made her say, "That's fine. I'll see you then."

That weekend was one of the last before Peregrine would go back to school. Even as they bounced over the rapids in their canoe, shouting commands at each other—"Left! No, ready—right!"—she was thinking of everything she had to do to prepare for the semester. The crashing of the water, the warmth of the sun on her skin, the wind cooling the sweat under her life vest—it was all lost to her. Finally, they reached a calm stretch of river and lay their oars down in the boat. Peregrine's muscles burned, and she leaned back on her elbows, tilting her face to the sky.

"See, Peregrine?" Andrew said, smiling. "It's not so bad, is it? Living here?"

"Mmm." Peregrine closed her eyes.

"I mean, I know it's not Paris," he went on, "but what's so bad about a simple life? Nice little house, couple of kids— I'll have my own business soon. You'll be a doctor. You can open a practice, and we'll be all set. It'd be perfect."

"Right."

"Let's get married."

Her eyes flew open. Andrew was staring at her earnestly. He shifted his weight on the boat and reached for her hand. "I don't have a ring or anything," he said, "but you know, once the business is up and running ... anyway. What do you say?"

She opened her mouth and then closed it again. Finally, she said, "Andrew, you *cannot* be serious. We're twenty years old. I'm not even out of school yet!"

"So? You can't finish if we get married? I'll move in with you. It'll be great!"

She laughed. "Andrew. Come on. I care for you, but no. Not now."

For a moment, they just looked at each other. Andrew's olive skin shone in the sun. His eyes were begging her. Finally, he pulled away. "Let's go back."

If Peregrine thought the conversation was over, she was dead wrong. Over the next few months, it seemed she and Andrew couldn't see or speak to each other without him asking her to marry him. It was *consuming* him—and figuring out how to escape it was consuming her.

"We can move to Paris," he tried one night in his truck. "I'll go anywhere with you. Just pick a place and we'll start a life."

"No, Andrew," she said. "I'm sorry. I can't."

Then, one night, he showed up at her apartment in tears.

He was shaking when he held her hands, and Peregrine guided him to the living room couch. He couldn't sit for more than a second before jumping back to his feet and pacing the floor. "You don't understand," he said. "You don't need anyone or anything, I get that, but I *need* you. I can't live without you. I won't, Peregrine. Do you hear what I'm saying?"

Peregrine watched him, this boy she'd known forever, in shock. Was he saying what she thought he was?

"I mean," he continued, shaking his head, "what's the point? Why should I even try if you won't marry me? There's nothing else out there for me."

"Andrew, you can do—"

"No!" He dropped down beside her and held her hands tightly. "I can't do anything without you. Please, Peregrine. You have to marry me. You have to."

Peregrine's chest burned. She could see the little boy she used to climb trees with when she looked into those green eyes. She could also see her future slipping away . . . along with her power, self-respect, and everything she'd learned about herself in Paris.

"Okay," she said. And with that four-letter word, she gave up the dream of her authentic life in sacrifice to another's need. She knew that many parts of her would die with this commitment, but what was the alternative?

. . .

"*What* are you talking about?" her father demanded when she went home the next weekend. Peregrine knew better than to break the news while Andrew was with her, so she picked a night when he was out with his buddies at a ballgame.

Peregrine's parents had married young, and both of them had often told her they wanted her to experience the world, date around, and wait to get married at least until she was done with college. But her parents loved Andrew, too, almost as a son. They knew he'd be trustworthy, steady, and loving. As unworldly as he was, he'd give the shirt off his back to a friend, so he'd probably lay down his life for their daughter.

"If you . . ." Peregrine's father started, then continued. "I will support you whatever you choose to do. But I wish you wouldn't. I really wish you wouldn't."

Peregrine's mother said nothing. They both knew that theirs wasn't a relationship in which her opinions would sway Peregrine one way or the other.

"Andrew needs me," she said simply.

In the winter of that year, Peregrine stood in a simple white dress in the back of her hometown church. She lightly gripped her father's arm, breathing deeply to calm her nerves.

Peregrine's father gently touched her chin to draw her attention to him. He looked into her eyes. "Sweetheart, I did the same thing you're doing. I've lived the effects for more than twenty years. Please—don't do this. Walk out of this church right now."

"Dad!" Peregrine exclaimed.

"I'll help you," her father said. "You can go wherever you want, start over, get away. Hell, you can come back and marry Andrew five years from now, but don't do it today!"

For a moment, Peregrine just stared into her father's kind, intense eyes. Then she shook her head. "There are two hundred people in there. I can't—I won't—leave him at the altar."

"You can," he urged her. "I know it will hurt him—"

"It would break his heart, Dad," Peregrine said. "And I will not do that to him. Somehow, I'm going to make this work." At the time she said the words, she believed them. She had convinced herself that maybe she could maintain a life of authenticity outside this arrangement. With that, the wedding march started playing on the church's sound system.

The ushers opened the door, Peregrine nodded at her dad, and the two of them strode down the thick red carpet toward Andrew. She felt like a passive participant as Andrew beamed at her from the front of the church. This wasn't her wedding; it was his. *Dear god*, she thought, *this is not right. How can I be doing this to myself? I'm settling. Am I really consciously making this choice?*

. . .

Andrew moved into her little one-bedroom apartment and hardly made a dent in the surroundings—except for the trash that he and his friends left after their beer-drinking sessions. When spring classes started back up, Peregrine switched to working for Mimi from seven to three and went to classes from four to ten. Andrew worked seven to three in a car repair shop (he was still applying for loans), and hung out with his old high school friends every night.

Peregrine's classes were a welcome escape from her life with Andrew. In class, she could lose herself in theories of brain chemistry and not think about this husband with whom she couldn't picture the future she had once dreamed. She ached with mixed emotions. After all, she did love Andrew as a friend; it wasn't as if he were a stranger or someone she despised. Yet, she was missing so much in this relationship: passion, creativity, sexuality, openness—parts of herself she knew existed because she had already experienced them. But those parts were drifting further and further away. At the same time, her commitment to Andrew was still stronger than the commitment to live the life she wanted. The only thing she could do to ease the conflict within her was attempt a positive shift in attitude about her life with him.

Andrew had taken college classes the previous year but dropped out, saying he was "too stupid for college." Peregrine told him over and over again what an amazing artist he was and how proud she was of him for his skills. He could draw anything and build anything with his hands, and he did start making a little money at his shop. Of course, it was hard to tell because he didn't keep up with his own books and didn't feel he was making enough to hire a bookkeeper.

Peregrine felt as though everything Andrew accomplished was only because she pushed or pulled him into doing it. She took care of everything in the household, from laundry to finances. How had she become just another mother to him? Why the hell did he seem to *need* a mother at his age? The idea was impossibly foreign to her—and, in the literal sense of the word, it was *exhausting* her. She emptied herself out on a daily basis to build him up without the support ever being returned. She was his life coach, while her own life slipped away. She was in this relationship yet ever so lonely.

Just like that, time passed. It was all she could do to just get through each day. Her life was focused on her to-do list; action by action, she moved forward, but the connection with herself that she had found in Paris was long gone; she had stopped seeing herself with pure love and so was no longer able to find inspiration around her. Even the simple things—the beauty of flowers blooming in the spring—were lost to her. It was as if her world had turned gray. Moments of pleasure were fleeting and not nearly as intense as they used to be, and she knew it was because she was not in alignment with what she wanted in her life. She was trapped, and she didn't know how to stop the cycle of complacency. She performed the duties that were expected of her, but where was the beauty in this life?

About a year into their marriage, Peregrine and Andrew were essentially leading separate lives. He had his friends, and just for something to do—something to keep her out of the house—Peregrine learned to shed some of her introversion to make new friends. Some of them were quirky and nerdy, some were purely study buddies, and others belonged to an international crowd. She particularly enjoyed the latter, because she could invoke Parisian sensibilities when she was with them, dressing up and letting herself pretend she was leading a different life. Few of her friendships were deep, but that was all right with Peregrine. Her home life was so heavy that she craved lightness wherever she could find it.

One morning, she woke suddenly to her stomach heaving. She clapped a hand to her mouth and rushed to the bathroom. Even as she threw up, she recognized that she didn't actually feel *sick*. Peregrine took inventory: she hadn't had a drop to drink the night before. Nobody she knew had the flu. She hadn't eaten anything unusual.

Oh, my god, I'm pregnant! Her stomach fell as she sat, stunned, and started to cry. After a few minutes, she pulled on a pair of sweatpants and left the house without waking Andrew, who was still snoring after a night out with his friends.

She bought a pregnancy test at the nearest drugstore and used it right there in the store bathroom. She breathed deeply as she waited for the results, stick in hand. Soon, the telltale second line appeared. "Damn it," she said quietly, tears rising to her throat.

Peregrine had never wanted children. It wasn't part of her dreams, even as a child. When other little girls stuffed the skirts of their Barbie dolls to "give them a baby," she chose to go play outside with her brothers instead. Lately, more and more of her old classmates were getting married and pregnant, not necessarily in that order, and none of them looked as if they were happy. They looked stuck, in a city and a circumstance that Peregrine had always sworn she would never choose for herself. Yet, she had chosen it. She'd made a decision based on fear (what would Andrew do to himself if she didn't marry him?), and her mistake was irrevocable. How had she let it get this far? How had she settled for a marriage without real passion, true intimacy, or an authentic connection? How would she ever get out, much less forgive herself for her choice? And now she was having a child.

Swiftly, chokingly, Peregrine fell into a depression. Not that Andrew noticed. Four weeks passed before Peregrine finally brought herself to tell him she was pregnant.

It was over breakfast, just before they dashed out the door for their jobs, when she said almost offhandedly, "I've got news. I'm pregnant."

Andrew knocked his chair down as he jumped up to hug her. He pulled back when he noticed her stiffness. "What? Aren't you happy about this?"

"No," Peregrine said. "This is not what I wanted now. The timing is not right." There was so much more she could have said, but already she was feeling that the more she spoke out loud, the more real it became. A part of her still hoped it wasn't true. She didn't have the energy anymore to keep Andrew—a grown child—afloat, much less an *actual* child.

Andrew's face fell. "Maybe you just haven't had time to get used to it."

Peregrine grabbed her bag. "I'll see you tonight."

As usual, they left the apartment and went their separate ways.

With time, Peregrine came to recognize that this was the fact of her life, and she had to live with this reality. Each day of her pregnancy was a new day to try to shift her attitude about her situation. Whether it was planned or not, *desired* or not, they were having a child, and each day she worked on finding an ounce of beauty in the idea of being a family. There was a hint of acceptance on the horizon. Maybe she could make this work. After all, there was a sweet new life growing within her that deserved to be born in all the love in the world.

About six months into her pregnancy, Peregrine noticed that Andrew was spending more evenings out of the apartment than hanging there with the boys. One night, she dreamed of him holding hands with another woman. When she awoke, she felt the weight of truth; it was too heavy for make-believe, and she had an amazing intuition when she decided to listen to it.

While bringing their morning eggs from the stove to the table, she looked at him straight in the eyes. "Andrew, I had this dream last night that you were cheating on me. Is there any truth to that?"

Andrew blinked. "Peregrine."

"Yes?"

He hung his head and was silent for a moment. In that moment, she had her answer. Without looking up at her, he said, "We were too young to get married. I wasn't ready."

"*You* weren't ready?" Peregrine cried. Her stomach turned, and the baby kicked inside her—from the outpouring of adrenaline or shock, she didn't know. She sat down quietly, looking at her own plate. "Jesus, Andrew," she said. "So you're having an affair."

"Yes. Peregrine—I'm sorry. It really doesn't mean anything. I do love you; it's just sex."

They stared at each other in silence. Peregrine's mind raced. She couldn't decide if she wanted to punch him in the face, cry hysterically, or throw up. *Here it is*, she thought. *My excuse to leave.* Relief poured through her, but along with it was anger—she'd married Andrew for *his* sake, not hers, and now he was claiming *he* wasn't ready? Then came sadness that there was a new life being born into the world, and it would enter into a broken home. The guilt was insurmountable. She could only blame Andrew so much. She'd gotten herself into this situation. Now the only question was how she could fix it. She knew it was her responsibility to take back control of her life.

Peregrine left the apartment, and the day passed in a blur of work and school. That night, no music from Andrew's stereo could be heard from outside the apartment. Peregrine sensed that he was waiting quietly inside to take his medicine, and she took a few minutes to herself before going in. Their marriage was over. That was the conclusion she had come to. She paused to assure herself it was the right choice. She would give it a few months after the baby was born, but after that, she was out of there.

Peregrine labored at home, pacing the floors for two days before heading to the hospital for her natural childbirth. She grabbed the bar on the hospital bed and pushed so long that her arms felt like jelly. Her body shook with effort and pain. Andrew was there the whole time, infinitely kind and patient with her. "You've got this," he soothed. "I'm so proud of you." Despite everything they'd been through, Peregrine was grateful for his presence in the room, for his solid warmth beside her and his help as she pushed and pushed through thirteen hours of labor. In his eyes, she could see the old friendship and love left on a shelf between them, and that gave her comfort.

When the baby—Alice—was born, Peregrine was so weak that she couldn't even hold her. With a tender smile, Andrew held Alice before her. Her heart squeezed when she looked at her daughter. It was a sensation of all-encompassing love, starting deep within Peregrine, filling her entirely, and radiating outward—toward Alice, toward Andrew, toward the world. Peregrine's eyes clouded with tears as she realized that *this*—exactly what she was experiencing—was true beauty. True beauty came from pure love. It was so obvious. There was nothing Peregrine wanted more than to sustain this feeling forever and to apply it to all aspects of her life. The only way to do that, she understood with stark clarity, was to return to living authentically, starting with pure love for herself. She hadn't been true to herself in so long, and she had compromised so much . . . what kind of example would that be for Alice? No—Peregrine needed to return to herself, a rejoining of her mind, body, and sprit. She had to make some changes deep within. There was no other way to reclaim her personal power. It all had to start with forgiveness.

Debrief

SEPARATION: YELLOW FLAME

The yellow flame illuminates your personal power. A point of joining body and mind, this flame doesn't just relate to physical power and strength—but to strength of mind. When the yellow flame burns brightly, it offers healthy self-worth, esteem, and confidence, giving us the power to constantly align ourselves with our unlimited potential. When the flame is dim, we are susceptible to moving away from what we seek. We are open to situations that do not serve our highest good, causing resentment for ourselves as well as others. Co-dependency often develops from this weak flame. In these types of relationships, we aren't free to walk our own paths. When we try to fix others' deficiencies, we take from them their opportunity to grow as human beings and find their own unlimited potential. Meanwhile, we rob ourselves of energy and set ourselves up for failure every time. We must walk our own paths!

To brighten this flame, we must realign ourselves with pure self-love, which cultivates the ability to see the pure love and unlimited potential for self, others, and the world at large. If we each tended to our own beautiful garden, the collective beauty in the world would be immeasurable.

What or who is the source of your power? ∾ Do you give control of your power to another and then ask for some of it back? ∾ Do you over-compromise? ∾ Do you excessively put others' needs before your own? ∾ Do you know what you truly desire? ∾ Do you live in alignment with that desire? Or do you constantly live outside that desire and then wonder why you experience negative thoughts and emotions? ∾ Are you co-dependent or in a co-dependent relationship? Are you an enabler? ∾ Are you worried about the future or in despair over your current situation? ∾ Are you facing your fears or ignoring them? Answering these questions is the start of activating the yellow flame within you.

CHAPTER 4

Green Flame: Hebrides Islands

GREEN FLAME: *The green flame illuminates the potential for love in its purest form—self-love. Through love for self, we are open to giving and receiving pure love outside ourselves. This flame also gives us the ability to see others are they really are: pure love.*

Shortly after Alice was born, Peregrine filed for divorce. Her separation from Andrew happened smoothly, amicably. They treated each other fairly and with respect, and he vowed to be as present in Alice's life as Peregrine would allow. She believed him because, against all odds, Andrew was an excellent father. Before the divorce, he never shied away from changing diapers, giving feedings, waking up at odd hours, or watching Alice when Peregrine had to be in school or work. Peregrine knew she could depend on him to love and protect Alice, and she was grateful. It allowed her to achieve her first major goal: dive intensely into her studies.

Quickly, Peregrine so impressed her advisor that he added her as a co-author to a project he was doing with other researchers at a university in Scotland. When it came time for the pair to go to Scotland to present their work, Peregrine took an extra ten days of vacation; since the university had paid for her flight and Alice was safe at home with Andrew, she thought it was the perfect time to see the Hebrides Islands—a place that supposedly embodied intense natural beauty.

"Peregrine, you wouldn't believe it. It's so far north, but the weather there is like the Caribbean," said Mimi, who had vacationed in the Hebrides several years earlier. Now in her eighties, Mimi was a bit more fragile, but the fire in her eyes was the same as Peregrine remembered from her childhood. "The beaches are beautiful, and the weather is warm and mild. You'll love it. And honey," Mimi added firmly, "you need a vacation."

Aside from the six weeks Peregrine had taken off right after Alice's birth, she hadn't given herself a vacation since Paris. So, after saying goodbye to her advisor in Edinburgh, she flew northwest across the mountain ranges to the Isle of Harris.

Looking out the plane window, she nearly gasped at the contrast between the deep moss-colored mountainsides, the dark rocks that cracked open the green and sparkled in sunlight, and the turquoise water. It was breathtaking. Peregrine felt a shock to the senses, an electrical reminder of the beauty in the natural world. She couldn't wait to see more, to bask in it.

Once she landed, Peregrine paid for a rental car and slid into what, back home, would be the passenger seat. "Here goes," she said out loud as she looked over her left shoulder to reverse.

Driving on the left side of the road was an interesting challenge. The scenery was so lovely that it was a little too easy for Peregrine's mind to wander and her vehicle to cross the center line. After catching herself a time or two, she shook her head and giggled at herself. There would be plenty of time for sightseeing when she out of the car, and she was sure that the other drivers on the road would appreciate her focus—especially when she reached the first of several traffic roundabouts. Circling the "wrong way" felt terribly reckless, even though she knew she was driving appropriately. Peregrine smiled. She was all too familiar with the feeling of "recklessly going around the wrong way." She was pleased at the lightness her heart found in that association.

Driving on the single road that traced the island, there was no way for Peregrine to miss the village where she'd rented a cottage. The cottages themselves almost disappeared from the road, as they were designed to blend into the hillside. Instead of a shingled or even thatched roof, the slightly rounded roofs were covered in grass, and the stone exterior walls looked almost like pieces of an ancient castle. The real beauty was the view of the ocean, and the cottages were designed to take full advantage: large wraparound windows took in a panoramic scene of the ocean to the west, and Peregrine couldn't wait for sunset. The tiny kitchen featured a U-shaped layout of burled wood cabinets topped with dark granite countertops. One quaint bedroom in the back held a welcome basket with a bottle of champagne—her favorite!—and local snacks of oat crisps, salmon, and shortbread cookies. There was a private sauna in the back room, with plenty of space, Peregrine noted, for a visiting massage therapist to set up her table. Best of all, there would be no Internet, no cell phone, and no interruptions from the outside world. Except for occasional check-in calls with Andrew, this would be ten days of answering to nobody. In other words: heaven.

Peregrine carried in her luggage and then arranged herself on the couch to enjoy the ocean view. The sun streamed in, and she stretched out like a cat. With her face and bare limbs warmed, she soon became drowsy and slipped into a dreamless sleep.

When she awoke, the sun had set and Peregrine's stomach reminded her of its emptiness. She recalled passing a little pub on her drive from the airport. Maybe she'd walk down, have a beer, and see what her dinner options might be.

The evening was mild, with a cool sea breeze that lifted the hem of Peregrine's light sweater as she walked. The island was tiny, quiet, and peaceful, and she wondered for a moment if the pub would even be open. The worry was unnecessary—lights shone as she approached, and laughter spilled out of open windows.

Mimi had told her, "There are no strangers to the people of the Celtic lands," and Peregrine had already experienced the friendliness of the Scots in Edinburgh, so she was unsurprised when the elderly barmaid cried in greeting. What *did* surprise her was how little she understood of the local dialect!

"Could I see a menu, please?" Peregrine ventured, afraid to answer what was obviously a question she couldn't decipher. The other pub patrons watched her with interest.

"Never mind me granny bletherin' about," said a waitress about Peregrine's age as she handed her the menu. "Are you stayin' in the cottages? If you need anythin', you come down here and ask for Rosie. That's me."

Peregrine grinned at Rosie. "Thanks for that," she said. "What's the best meal in the house?"

"That depends. Are you wantin' what the locals eat or the tourists?"

Peregrine looked around at the people inhabiting the pub. They all seemed healthy and strong. No waifs in the lot, nor was anyone as overweight as they might be in a similar bar back home. "What would you recommend?" she asked with a smile.

"Well, we eat lots of fish from the sea and lamb from the local farms, of course. And Granny is a pretty good cook of either one."

"How about lamb chops, then? And this mashed apples and potatoes dish sounds good."

"Me pleasure."

As soon as Rosie disappeared into the kitchen with the menu, a bearded man came by Peregrine's table with a broad smile and coarse hands, gifting her with a glass of beer. His grin showed crooked, slightly yellowing teeth, and his words were entirely unintelligible. Like a magician, Rosie reappeared out of nowhere with a basket of rolls. She bumped him with her hip. "Scat, nyaff, and let her alone to eat her dinner!" Leaving the bread and a dish of fresh, creamy yellow butter, Rosie headed back to the kitchen again. She called back over her shoulder to the chastised man and his friends, "I'll be right back, so leave this girl be!"

As on her trip to Paris, Peregrine was in a place where nobody knew her or her story, where she could simply "be" and not perform to anyone's expectations. So who did she want to be here? Which part of herself did she want to find? She thought about this as she dug into her delicious, filling lambchop meal. The words that kept coming to mind were "calm" and "love." She wanted to access the overwhelming sense of love she'd felt at Alice's birth, as well as the calm, centered part of herself that had disappeared in the life she'd led with Andrew.

After dinner, Peregrine walked back to her cottage. The sounds of crashing waves echoed in the dark all around her. There was such force and power behind the breaking of the surf, and it made Peregrine feel at peace to realize that the ocean, the rocks, and the fragrant heather on the hillside would be here even if she weren't. The existence of nature was independent of human participation, even though nature sometimes seemed to put on its beautiful show as if it were on stage.

The salty, clean scent of the sea lingered on Peregrine's skin and hair even after a hot shower. She smiled, breathing deeply, as she burrowed beneath a light down blanket. With a delicious feeling of freedom, she stretched out in bed, soaking up the coolness of the mattress. This bed was hers alone. She could start living for herself again. As that thought settled, Peregrine once again fell into a deep and contented sleep.

In the morning, she was drawn back to the beach as if by a magnet. She sat cross-legged on the sand, which was already warm under her legs and open palms. For several long minutes, she looked out at the ocean. Faraway fishing boats peppered the water, tiny dots of white on the vast blue. *I've been so busy, so angry, so focused on Alice and Andrew and my studies,* Peregrine thought. *But look at this place. Look at this world. I haven't been paying attention.*

Peregrine couldn't deny there was something bigger than herself in the world. Not just the sea and the earth, of course, but a whole natural *system* she could hardly comprehend. As she watched the waves, as majestic as Mimi had promised, Peregrine thought of individual cells within a body, each one performing exactly the action it was meant to do. The rhythmic movement of the ocean seemed to echo the rhythms of her heart and breath. Everything was intertwined.

"Four seconds in," she said quietly. "Six seconds out."

Breathing was something she had learned in a college yoga class: each inhalation should be through the nose, slow and steady for four seconds. After a slight easy pause, the breath should be released through the mouth for six seconds. Breath was the first step in meditation. It had the ability to be detoxifying as well as invigorating. Seagulls called over the breaking surf, and a light breeze lifted the hair from her neck.

Four seconds in, she thought. *Six seconds out.*

Despite the attempted focus, her mind kept wandering home. Andrew had always been good with Alice, but was he feeding her at the right times? Was he dropping her off at Mimi and Grandpa's house when he promised?

Four seconds in.

There were still things of his in her apartment—his hiking

boots and last load of laundry, their high school yearbook that he insisted on keeping. When was he going to pick them up? Their divorce had gone through months ago.

Six seconds out.

Her old hurt and disappointment bubbled to the surface. How could she have married him? That *feeling*, walking down the aisle. No excitement. Only the chest-tightening knowledge that she was making the wrong choice even as she made it. How could she have married somebody who would threaten to hurt himself if she left him? How could she have prioritized *his* life, *his* happiness, so completely over her own?

Four seconds in.

People had to take their own path. That was what she'd learned. Peregrine's acceptance of the caretaking role had actually hindered Andrew's growth and done them *both* a disservice. Mistakes all around. Peregrine sighed gustily and opened her eyes. Meditation was harder than she'd thought it would be, but she was determined to master it. She needed to learn how to calm her mind.

Back in her cottage, Peregrine sifted through a menu of brochures on the coffee table. Golf, kite surfing, archery— no, no, no at least not that day. The deluxe honeymoon massage package? Could she get that for one? She needed a honeymoon with herself! There were no brochures for a meditation teacher, but Peregrine suspected the masseuse could point her in the right direction. She picked up the phone and called the number, setting up an appointment for that afternoon.

In the meantime, she changed into shorts and a casual top

and rolled out the bicycle supplied with her cottage rental. In the soothing sunshine, she adjusted it for her height and set off for an hour of exploring the nearby villages.

. . .

Later that day, the masseuse's efforts practically put Peregrine in a trance. A vigorous, full-body sea salt scrub made Peregrine feel she was shedding skin cells like a snake—but along with the skin cells, she started to feel released from the shackles of self-contempt she'd placed on herself in the last two years.

"This scrub is my personal blend," said Lucia, the masseuse. "Rosemary for cleansing and rebalancing your energies, lemon balm for calming, and sage for energizing you again. It's all natural, all grown or acquired here. Even the sea salts come from our fine North Sea."

"Why is that important to you?" Peregrine asked. "Everything being natural and local?"

"Our bodies benefit from being one with the environment," Lucia said. "Think about how people used to live before cars and planes let them go wherever they wanted; they had to rely off what the earth gave them locally, and their bodies became accustomed to those resources. Why would somebody who lives here in Scotland want to use products made on the other side of the world? They won't work as well. Local use of resources—food, water, herbs—is like feeding your body from its creator."

Peregrine let out her breath in a long sigh as Lucia worked. "That does make sense," she murmured.

After the scrub, Lucia helped her rise from the table and

into the shower adjacent the sauna. "You let all that wash down the drain, and imagine that all the toxins, negative thoughts, and discouragement you have stored in your body are carried away by that salt. Step out cleansed. You are starting anew . . . I'll get the massage table ready again."

When Peregrine returned with a long, luxurious bath sheet wrapped around her, Lucia had fitted the table with clean sheets and warmed blankets. Lucia held the blanket up and turned her face away, discreetly screening Peregrine as she dropped her towel and lay face-up on the table.

"I suggest we do the massage in silence," Lucia said softly. "Talking can take you out of your body too much to fully appreciate the massage. As thoughts arise, rather than speaking them or even following them in your mind, imagine with each exhalation that you're blowing them out into a bubble that will rise in the air and drift away. Don't trouble yourself with them or berate yourself for having thoughts; just acknowledge them, thank them, and watch them float away. You are not attached to them. Use your breath to move them out, feel the sensations in your body, and simply be here now."

Be here now, Peregrine thought. "Oh, I—"

Smiling, Lucia tapped a finger to her lips, reminding Peregrine to try silence for a while.

The first thought Peregrine exhaled into an imaginary bubble was, "Be here now." As Lucia began working her magic on Peregrine's tight shoulders, Peregrine imagined various bubbles that housed words such as *fear, anger*, and *guilt* leaving her body and floating away, toward the shore and beyond. She had an image of the caterpillar in *Alice in Wonderland* sitting on the mushroom and blowing letters out of smoke. As in the story, her words seemed to disfigure to unreadable as they broke up in the atmosphere.

When the massage was complete, Lucia placed one hand on Peregrine's shoulder. "You can rest here as long as you like, and I'll wait on the couch."

Peregrine was so relaxed that she'd fallen deeply asleep midway through the massage and had forgotten were she left off with the bubbles. Comfortably wrapped in a robe, she found Lucia sitting before two fine china teacups filled with steaming, aromatic herbal teas.

"Oh, I thought you might nap awhile longer," Lucia said. "Your muscles were so tight—I've never seen a woman with shoulders so wrought with tension."

"That massage was amazing," Peregrine said. "I'm also trying to learn more about meditation. I thought maybe you could help if you have some time?"

Lucia smiled and sat back, handing the second teacup to Peregrine. "I have time. You were my last appointment today, and my child is being well cared for at her father's house."

"I have a daughter, too," Peregrine said. For some reason, offering that fact made her feel vulnerable. "She's also with her father. But you seem so calm and centered as you're working, whereas I feel like I've been a mess lately. How are you able to keep a balance?"

"Ah, 'calm and centered.' Well, I work at it," Lucia explained. "Meditation is a practice. I do it at least once daily, and I make sure the food my daughter and I eat is good, living food from the earth, mainly from here in Scotland. Getting enough rest is imperative, and that can be very hard with little ones. But teaching my daughter to meditate has helped with that, for both of us."

"How old is your daughter?"

Lucia smiled. "She's eleven. I started teaching her to quiet her thoughts when she was five, starting kindergarten. Young ones can meditate, and it works much more quickly for them. They learn quickly and can settle themselves just as fast once they know how. They gain the transformative effects quicker than adults, too. They have less to let go of, I think, and that helps."

Peregrine thought about that for a moment. She wondered how meditation might have served her if she'd learned at a younger age. It might be something to try with Alice, once she got older.

Lucia sipped her tea. "Now, considering how hard and tight your muscles were when we started, tell me: how is it that you, a twenty-three-year-old little mama, are here without your husband and baby?"

Peregrine sighed. "That is a long and unhappy story. Alice is nearly a year old, and I divorced her father about six months ago. He's a great dad, but he was a terrible husband—for me, at least. We just weren't right for each other. My daughter is wonderful, too, but I would feel smothered if I were with her all the time."

"For a lot of women, having a baby re-centers their life," Lucia said. "It's as though, before they became a mom, they were their own star, with their own gravity and way of moving through the world, and then once they have a child, the child becomes the star and the mom cycles in orbit around that star. It works for some but not for all."

"Does that *ever* work?" Peregrine replied. "Isn't that how moms end up self-medicating with wine and Xanax? It just seems like living entirely for your children leaves you with no boundaries or sense of self."

"Everyone needs and deserves a sense of self," Lucia said. "Many allow the loss, yes, but having children or a partner needn't extinguish your identity; it should add to it. It's a creator of contrast that leads to individual growth, and if you can manage that growth, you can provide a great example to your children as well."

Although Peregrine thought she was fully relaxed from the spa treatment, even more stress dropped away as Lucia spoke. She felt as if she could breathe more freely and deeply than she had in years. How could she not have noticed what her body had been trying to tell her with her tight muscles and shortness of breath? How could she have been so disconnected from the simplest, purest form of beauty: physical health?

Peregrine left Lucia with a promise to return at least once more before leaving the Hebrides. Already, she felt the start of becoming a new woman—or perhaps it was a return to the woman she'd left behind in Paris.

. . .

Peregrine spent much of her remaining time on the island doing yoga, journaling, and writing out concrete goals. She thought carefully about these goals. They needed to be authentic—things she *truly* wanted to achieve and things that were actionable. On a notepad, she wrote:

Work on my physical health: exercise, natural and local foods, relaxation

Learn how to "be here now"—practice meditation

Reconnect with myself as a woman

Forgive myself for veering off my path

Exemplify a mother who exhibits individualism and freedom to be herself

Regain alignment to my true self . . . unconditional self-love.

This last goal was the one that made Peregrine feel released of a great weight: unconditional self-love. *If I can love myself as fiercely and unconditionally as I love Alice, it will be impossible to compromise again.* The realization was shocking in its simplicity.

In meditation, Peregrine used Lucia's technique of letting imaginary bubbles carry away her thoughts. As her mind emptied, she found herself noticing so much more about the natural environment surrounding her and relating it to what she needed to do within herself. *We* are *nature,* she thought. *We're not a separate entity from the earth. We're made from the same elements; we depend on what the earth gives us to sustain our life. We need to honor the cycles of nature, hibernating or going where it's warm in wintertime, conserving our energy after long cycles of growth and effort. We are made up of a mind, body, and spirit; they are intertwined and inseparable. The key to living beautifully is to cultivate health in all aspects of self. This,* Peregrine thought, smiling, *is our philosopher's stone.*

On her last full day in the Hebrides, Peregrine rounded a curve on foot to see another pub with a view of the water. She ordered a gin and tonic and then seated herself at a small table outside. Relaxing in the sun, Peregrine gasped when she saw a little community of sea otters playing in the water and on the beach. Was anyone else seeing this? She looked around; it seemed she was the only one outside. Completely obliviously, the otters were performing just for her, and Peregrine's cheeks soon hurt from smiling. Watching them have so much fun simply *being* taught her an important lesson: she wanted to *live* vivaciously, carefree, and playfully, seeing the beauty in the world instead of all the tragedies. It was a conscious shift of attitude. She needed to give herself permission to move on from the experience of making such a compromising decision with Andrew. It was over and done, and she'd made it through. To love herself meant to forgive herself.

Debrief

CONJUNCTION: GREEN FLAME

The green flame begs the awakening of pure love within the self and is meant to restore wisdom, faith, harmony, and unity. Old beliefs, paths, and attitudes break down as the green flame lights the way down the path to renewal. This path is an opportunity leading to new awakenings: the building blocks for rebirth into pure love, acceptance, and forgiveness. Here, find permission to be gentle with yourself and to reestablish the connection to your soul, to heal from past transgressions and release negative and harmful thoughts so that health of mind, body, and spirit can be restored. Finding love for ourselves should be a priority at the top of the list because without this self-love, we cannot give or receive love from others.

The green flame is the master of transmutation for beauty, enhancing love, compassion, and oneness with nature (from which we are not separate). If the green flame had a descriptor, it would be joy, and when it burns brightly, the giving and receiving of love knows no bounds. This is where unconditional love is born. We want to live in joy and know we have moved from alignment with our true beings when we experience feelings outside of joy.

What is your understanding of unconditional love? ❧ Are you struggling to accept yourself as you are? ❧ Do you have destructive thoughts about yourself or someone else? ❧ Do you have enough self-love to understand the concept of love for others?

CHAPTER 5

Blue Flame: Colorado

BLUE FLAME: *Your truth will set you free! The blue flame enhances the wisdom of your mind, body, and spirit and allows you to outwardly express this beauty with the world.*

Peregrine returned home from the Hebrides refreshed and rejuvenated. Her skin was glowing from the natural scrubs and lotions she'd been using—and the natural, local foods she'd eaten—smiles came more easily and more often, and the light of her heart seemed to shine through her eyes. Mimi saw the change as soon as Peregrine arrived to pick up Alice. "Now *this* is the Peri I know," she said with a fierce embrace. "I missed her."

Peregrine had missed her, too.

She spent the afternoon with Mimi, connecting and catching her up on her travels. Mimi listened with a smile, living vicariously through Peregrine's stories.

"I am so happy and proud of the transformation you seem to be making," Mimi said. "As I have always known, there is so much more to you than what others can see, but now you're letting your light shine."

Unlike when she'd returned from Paris, Peregrine held on to the realizations she'd made and the goals she'd set. As a tribute to her physical health, she ransacked her pantry and cabinets, throwing out any food that was boxed or bagged. She started shopping for local, organic food and beauty products and practiced meditation daily. The largest change, however, came from unconditional self-love. She evaluated each decision in her life by asking herself whether her choice was in alignment with loving herself; did it bring her joy? Understanding that her true self wanted to stay in alignment with joy, she used other emotions as a guidance system that she was veering from that alignment. She found that when she let joy guide her, she set firmer boundaries and remained on a path that felt positive and beautiful—even if it wasn't what she expected.

Peregrine took and scored well on her MCATs and gained acceptance into a prestigious medical school. But something was nagging at her. When she thought about starting medical school in several months, she didn't feel excited or happy. She felt a sense of tiredness, of quiet dread, that was *not* in alignment with joy. Though she knew her family would object, she decided to put off med school for a year. She needed to push the pause button before she made another major decision. She needed a change, some distance. She needed a move.

Decision made, Peregrine felt instantly as if a heavy weight had been lifted. She started investigating job options online and soon found an opportunity in the beautiful mountains of Colorado as a controller of a historic hotel that was being renovated. With years of experience working at Mimi's accounting firm, Peregrine was confident she could do the job. Sure enough, her phone interview ended with an invitation for an on-site interview and tour.

Colorado was breathtaking. The cornflower blue skies were uninterrupted through the windshield of Peregrine's rental car, and the snow-peaked mountains were a stunning backdrop for a Southern girl accustomed to flat soggy deltas. The sheer natural beauty of her surroundings reminded Peregrine of the Hebrides, though the landscape was entirely different.

The hotel was a short distance from the ski mountain, and while its exterior was intact, the inside was gutted. Walls had been torn down, and the floors were all open spaces, exposed wires, and HVAC ducts. The carpet had been pulled up to reveal bare concrete floors. Peregrine imagined what it could look like after the renovation—wood and stone floors, warm-colored walls, cozy fireplaces. She was attracted to the space and hoped the hotel developer wouldn't be too distracted about her college degree being in such an unrelated field. The fact that her interview occurred during the tour itself was a little surprising to Peregrine, who was expecting to sit across a desk from the man, but it ended with the words she wanted to hear: "How soon can you start?"

Peregrine's heart pounded. "Well, I'd have to pack everything, find a place, and get my daughter ready to come out, so . . . six weeks? Is that soon enough?"

"How about if I give you a head start on finding a place?" The developer pulled a business card from his pocket, explaining that an acquaintance was moving to London but was not yet ready to sell his house. "It's an easy commute to the hotel, and I gather there are good schools in that neighborhood. If it works out, maybe you could move here by the end of the month?"

Peregrine agreed and contacted the acquaintance right away. She followed the directions he gave her on the phone and soon pulled up to a garage at the bottom of a three-story contemporary structure. The house was set in the side of what felt like a mountain to Peregrine (though she later learned it was "just a foothill"). There, she got her first lesson in mountain architecture: it was so expensive to excavate that most builders constructed duplexes instead of single-family homes to make the construction cost-effective.

The duplex was a "contemporary lodge" design: exposed beams, an elk antler chandelier, and wide plank flooring. The kitchen and living room, one floor up from the garage downstairs, had enormous windows overlooking the city down in the valley. The bedrooms were another level above, and the master bedroom offered the same view from a slightly different angle. Both the living room and the bedroom levels had wraparound decks, and she could envision evenings enjoying the sunset. Since she and Alice had the habit of sharing a bed, the second, smaller bedroom would be a good playroom. She could drive out a truck with her furniture, and the mix of her antiques with the house's more modern architecture would be eclectic and interesting in a different way than her apartment in the French Quarter. Peregrine's intuition told her that she and Alice could be happy here. That was all she needed to know. After a quick meeting with the homeowner, they sealed the deal with a handshake. As soon as she could get everything packed up in New Orleans, she and Alice would be heading for a brand new adventure in Colorado. She was ready to take this leap of faith, *moving*—not just traveling—to a location where no one knew her name. It was time to work on rising from the ashes.

. . .

By the time Peregrine arrived for her first day at work, construction workers filled the building. She spent a good part of her days running up and down the six flights of stairs to get signatures and approval on paperwork and check on progress in different parts of the property. Soon she was filing for permits, supervising the contractors, and selecting carpets and other fixtures. Working seven days a week, she broke out of her shell to schmooze all the people who made things happen in this little mountain town, from city employees through managers of other hotels. With cultivated confidence, it wasn't long before she was making more money than the job had advertised but with a *lot* more responsibility.

Each morning and evening, she gave herself a chance to breathe by sitting outside on her porch swing. She was intentional about not allowing her work life to steal her appreciation for the beauty of her surroundings. In the mornings, she witnessed the most beautiful sunrises casting shadows into the valley, and in the evenings, she gazed at the twinkling lights in the town below her. Sunsets lingered, the sky turning from blue to blood-orange before drowsily settling back into a deep, rich sapphire. Some nights, storms rolled through from the west, and Peregrine watched them from her higher perch. Where she sat, the skies were clear and blue. It was like she was already living in the future, when the storms had ended. *How strange*, she thought. If you were down in the valley, you had no idea when the rain would end, and no clue that—somewhere above you—it had never even begun. Peregrine was enamored by what felt like an apt metaphor for life: *blue sky always exists above the storms.* She was so grateful to be above the clouds these days.

The downside to the mountain air, however, was that Peregrine's skin was starting to relate to the alligators in the Lubriderm commercials. Moving from a humid, southern climate to the dry, high altitudes of Colorado was a shock for her system. The mountains were gorgeous and the air was bracing, but she had completely dried up. She had to stop wearing her contact lenses and switch back to glasses, her skin was dry and cracked, her nose bled frequently, and her throat was always scratchy. Even carrying around a gallon jug of water and refilling it constantly didn't help; she felt dehydrated all the time. It seemed she just couldn't replenish her skin's moisture, and creams and lotions didn't help. Then a friend of hers from work suggested that she visit the natural cave saunas.

An hour away from town was the world's largest natural hot springs and system of underground cave saunas. The waters were loaded with minerals, and people traveled from all over the country to experience their healing properties. Maybe that was what her skin needed. Something directly from nature instead of from a bottle.

One weekend, with arrangements made for Alice to have

a play date with a school friend, Peregrine drove out to the springs. She certainly wasn't the only one with the idea. Locals and vacationers alike populated the springs, sinking deep into the warm waters and closing their eyes in bliss. Peregrine wandered away from the more crowded areas. The natural pools within the caves gave her the deep relaxation of a hot tub—with a slight earthy scent of sulfur instead of chlorine—lovely humid air to breathe, and the smooth sensation of her skin drinking up what it needed. The caves reminded her of the movies she used to watch with Mimi—all mysterious darkness with more than a hint of creepiness. Now, as then, Peregrine revisited the feeling that she was exploring the unknown.

After a few trips to the springs, Peregrine noticed her back reddening. From far away, it looked like a mild sunburn. She used a hand mirror to examine it more closely in her bathroom mirror and winced. From this perspective, it was clearly a rash, stretching angrily between her shoulder blades. By the following day, it had spread up to the nape of her neck. A day after that, the redness reached down past the hem of her shirt. Peregrine was officially concerned.

"Does it hurt?" Alice asked from the bathroom doorway.

Peregrine handed Alice the aloe vera spray she'd been using. "Like you wouldn't believe," she said. "Spray me, would you?"

Over the next week, the rash intensified to look like bad acne—red bumps peaked with white tips. Peregrine was horrified. Was she actually in an episode of *The Twilight Zone*? She had never seen anything like this before! She made an appointment with a dermatologist and, just in case, stopped wearing the signature scent she'd developed in Paris. She also sought out hypoallergenic, fragrance-free soaps, shampoo, and lotions. Nothing helped. Not even the dermatologist Peregrine visited could figure out the problem, and not a single cream he prescribed made any difference. As the weather warmed, Peregrine looked with longing at the halter tops in her closet. No way was she wearing anything that would reveal this rash to the world. Instead, she wore high-necked, long blouses to cover the condition. Though no one could see it but her, Peregrine felt more self-conscious than she ever had about her physical state of beauty. She knew the only way to restore her confidence in her external beauty was to bring back her health from within . . . she just didn't know how.

One day at work, the friend who had recommended the springs noticed Peregrine was more fidgety than usual. "What's up?" Paisley asked.

"This rash is driving me insane! I feel like an extra in *Tales From the Crypt!*"

"The rash from the caves?" Paisley asked, surprised. "Wasn't that six months ago?"

Peregrine nodded miserably.

"Look. I know my last suggestion didn't exactly pan out, but you have to call my acupuncturist." Paisley pulled out her cell and texted a number to Peregrine. "It won't be treatment you're used to, but I'm sure he'll be able to help. I was diagnosed with fibromyalgia a few years back, and he helped me completely get rid of the pain."

Peregrine took the card, willing herself to hold it with both hands so she wouldn't scratch. No matter the temperature, her skin felt hot to the touch. The sensation when she scratched was like rubbing the edge of an ice cube over her skin, followed immediately by a burning deep in her muscle tissue. Once she scratched one spot, even just a little, the rest of her back demanded similar attention. "Thanks," she said, unconvinced. "I'll give it a try."

At this point in her life, Peregrine's exposure to natural healing and herbal medicines was minimal. She knew of no acupuncturists back home and, without realizing it, had internalized feelings that it wasn't "real" medicine. At the same time, her experiences in Scotland had awakened her to a new way of looking at healing. She had vowed to bring that openness to nature home with her, so she made an appointment.

The acupuncturist's office was painted and decorated in soothing, spa-like shades of blue and brown. His intake was long and exhausting; as Peregrine talked about her itching and pain, the acupuncturist asked more questions to refine the details. Soon he was asking about her menstrual cycle, her diet here, her diet back in New Orleans, and how much sleep she got on a typical night. She couldn't imagine these things were relevant, but something about his tone and language made her sense that the questions were important, so she continued to answer.

Finally, he said, "You have a build-up of toxic heat in your system."

"Toxic heat?" Peregrine's eyebrows furrowed skeptically. "What's that? I've never heard of it."

"It's a build-up of heat in the body from defense against an external pathogen," he explained. "I think you've picked up a fungal infection from the cave or the springs. Naturally, that means no more caves for a while. Also, stay away from spicy foods. Eat yogurt and fresh vegetables instead," he continued, writing down his suggestions. "Practice the quiet asanas of yoga daily, and avoid inversions. I'll send you home with some herbs that you make into tea to drink every day."

The acupuncturist then gave Peregrine an envelope of bath tea to soak in, advising her to make sure she cleaned her bathtub first and afterward with non-chlorine bleach. Before she left, he gave her an acupuncture treatment to give her some relief until the herbs kicked in. To Peregrine's surprise, the needles didn't hurt. The experience was oddly meditative, almost trance-like, and she actually did feel better afterward.

At home, although the acupuncturist's regimen made Peregrine feel as if she'd moved from a swamp monster movie into a *Harry Potter* sequel, she followed his directions precisely. Every morning, she sipped the ghastly tea, which eventually didn't taste as terrible as it did the first time. In the evenings, while watching the storms roll past, she drank her second tea.

Within six weeks of the acupuncture, diet, and lifestyle regimen, ninety percent of her skin condition had cleared. After another six weeks, the skin not only on her back but also her face and hands was pristine, silky-smooth, and beautiful again. A little voice inside her was tempted to declare her recovery a matter of "time healing all wounds" more than the alternative interventions, but her larger self was putting the pieces together: it was nature that had healed her when Western medicine couldn't.

If she wasn't already convinced, she soon had a snow-boarding accident and dislocated her shoulder. After putting the shoulder back in place, the emergency room doctors couldn't do much more for the pain than give her some pills and a sling, so she returned to the acupuncturist. As he "needled" her, Peregrine felt herself relaxing into the mental state she usually achieved at the end of her yoga sessions.

"Chinese meridians closely mimic the neurological pathways that run through your body," he explained afterward. "When working with pain disorders, we can utilize these pathways to affect how the brain receives pain signals from the injured area. It also has a profound effect on the localized area of injury by stimulating circulation, which helps heal the damaged muscles more quickly."

That was it. From her skin disorder to her dislocated shoulder, Peregrine had become a believer.

. . .

When Alice's school let out for the summer, Peregrine arranged with the airline for Alice to fly back to New Orleans to stay with Andrew for six weeks. In the meantime, Peregrine sought out some extracurricular activities of her own.

First on her agenda was to learn more about Colorado's regional plants and herbs—specifically, their medicinal and healing properties. Peregrine's experience with the acupuncturist had lit a new flame of curiosity within her, especially because it seemed to echo what Lucia had said in the Hebrides about local resources being the healthiest. Why *did* Peregrine so often first turn to pharmaceuticals to cure her ills? Why did most people? They certainly had their place, but maybe they shouldn't be the first choice. She thought about the old apothecaries and some modern chemists in Europe; there, pharmacists commonly compounded, or made customized medications, to suit people's unique needs using herbals or homeopathic remedies. This, too, seemed miles ahead of Western medical beliefs, which sent people to collect mass-produced medications without regard for their unique body compositions and health issues. *Sometimes*, she thought, *the old ways are the best ways.*

After doing a little research, Peregrine signed up for a series of nature walks geared toward those interested in Western herbalism. A friendly, open-faced guide in a floppy hat led the class of five students. Together, they set off on a mountainside trail populated with plants that, to Peregrine, initially all looked the same. The guide stopped the group every so often, pointing out horsemint and wormwood sage, asking them to bend low to the ground and rub their fingers against the plant stems.

"Smell that?" he asked as he deeply inhaled the aroma of the sage. "Such a lovely, fresh scent, isn't it? This is a great plant that can be used for digestive disorders, menstrual cramps, or even sprains."

Peregrine looked with interest at what she would have considered a fairly nondescript, even weed-like plant. The leaves were silky against her fingers, and the guide was right about the freshness of the smell; it reminded her of the Thanksgiving table. She could imagine this tasting good in some kind of tea.

The walk continued for almost two hours, time that passed quickly with the guide's knowledgeable instruction about each plant, including how to grow, harvest, and store the dried herbs. He was enthusiastic about teaching practical uses for the herbs, and his love for nature, plants, and herbs was palpable.

Toward the end of the day, the guide noticed Peregrine scratching at her legs. "Bug bites?" he asked sympathetically.

"Always." Peregrine shook her head. "I should have thought to bring some Off with me."

The guide laughed. "Haven't you learned anything today? Look, come here."

He gestured her under the shade of a large ponderosa tree while the rest of the class watched. "See these?" He knelt down and squinted up at Peregrine as he touched a light lavender-colored flower. "This is the sticky purple geranium. The flowers are actually edible, but *you* might be interested in the leaves—they serve as a nice antihistamine."

Peregrine laughed, realizing how impulsively she thought of over-the-counter treatments. "Well, let's put it to the test."

She bent down and copied the guide's motions as he reached around sharp areas of the stem to grasp the leaves. Gently, she rubbed the sticky plant against her bug bites. A sweet breeze cooled the gel-like substance, and she felt almost immediate relief of the itch. Just as suddenly, the sun emerged from behind a cloud, warming the skin that had just been cooled. It was as if a switch flipped inside Peregrine: the moment felt like a gift from nature. She didn't know whether to describe it as a moment of mental or spiritual transformation, but she suddenly knew with clarity that nature could provide whatever she needed if she intentionally made the effort to connect with it.

"It worked," she said quietly.

The guide grinned. "Well, what did you expect?"

. . .

After her experiences with acupuncture and the series of nature walks, Peregrine felt she was on the beginning of a new journey—but she didn't know the destination. All she could do was to listen to her body's communication. What brought her joy? What made her feel in alignment with her true self? What *didn't*? It was much easier to make decisions that kept her on her path when she was listening to her body—the things that made her feel light and energized were worth pursuing, while the ones that made her feel tired or made her shoulders and neck ache probably weren't doing her any good.

Not entirely to her surprise, Peregrine found she was happiest when she followed the path she had started with acupuncture and a more natural lifestyle. In the warm months, she kayaked, hiked, ran, and bicycled. In the cold months, she skied and snowboarded. Yoga and meditation were year-round, and Peregrine cooked using whole, organic, local ingredients. She also returned for regular acupuncture appointments, always engaging the acupuncturist in conversation about the field. The more she learned, the more she wanted to learn.

Alice, too, was thriving in this new lifestyle. Healthy and active, she made good grades and better friends, and Peregrine felt proud of the example she was providing. She saw with clarity that the lessons she'd learned in the Hebrides were now a part of her—a practiced, intentional part—and they were strengthened by what she was learning now: how to communicate the things that fulfilled her. She didn't worry about what anyone else, including her family, thought of her lifestyle. And she didn't hesitate to talk about her fascination with acupuncture and natural beauty with others, even those who might not understand. She brushed off critical comments from her mother as easily as the playing otters flipped water off their backs. Discarding fear of judgment was addictively liberating, and it attracted people into her life who were in alignment with her values. As a result, her friendships were harmonious, and she enjoyed a more fulfilling dating life than she ever had before.

As Peregrine's months in Colorado blended into years, she realized she was doing herself one major disservice: staying at job for which she felt no passion. Work was something she did to pay the bills, to do the things she truly enjoyed, but it wasn't what she envisioned for her future. It also was also another message she did not want to send to Alice. She didn't want to love *parts* of her life; she wanted to *live* in pure love for life, and that had to include her career. She had realized a new passion that could take her life in a more satisfactory route; she had to find out more.

Following her acupuncture appointment one afternoon, Peregrine asked, "How did you learn to do all this? Where did you go to school?"

He smiled. "I've noticed for a long time that your interest in acupuncture is more like a student than a patient. Are you considering a change?"

Peregrine gathered her bag from a chair and jewelry

from a small silver bowl. "More than considering it," she said. "I was supposed to go to med school, but it doesn't feel right anymore. I can't help but think that's my *old* path, and continuing down it would take me where I've already been, not where I want to go."

The acupuncturist took a card from his pocket and wrote the name of a website on the back. "Your spirit of curiosity would thrive in acupuncture school." He smiled as he handed it to her. "And Chicago is a great city."

Debrief

FERMENTATION: BLUE FLAME

The blue flame is the illuminator of our communication and outward expression of our authentic selves. It embodies elements of the red flame (identity), orange flame (sexuality/creativity), yellow flame (personal power), and green flame (unconditional love) to let us express our intimate truths, creative desires, and personal aspirations. Once this communication is released, manifestation can occur—thus the saying, "Watch your thoughts, for they become words; watch your words, they become actions." When this flame burns dimly, we are unable to express our true selves. Something is suppressing our outward communication, whether that is fear, disconnection from our spiritual selves, or social conditioning.

The blue flame is critical to living our most authentic, beautiful lives. It is the point of true liberation, when a balanced blend of intuition and personal wisdom allows us to ask for what we want and successfully communicate who we really are. This flame also acts as a bridge to the next flame levels, which illuminate and strengthen the spiritual parts of ourselves.

List the truths of your mind, body, and sprit: are you feeding your body with the best nutrition and fueling it with exercise? ✑ Are you listening to its communication? ✑ What about your mind? ✑ Are you communicating constructively with others? Or are you ignoring your internal guidance, compromising your feelings and beliefs to pacify others? ✑ Are you cultivating your spiritual self? ✑ What practices can you incorporate into your life to help you connect with your higher thoughts and vibrations? ✑ What fears or obstacles are you still hiding behind? ✑ How can you cultivate and communicate more beauty in the world?

CHAPTER 6

Violet Flame: Chicago

VIOLET FLAME: *This is the key flame in order to reach the pearlescent flame. It is the cleanser flame that prepares the lesser material of old mistakes and negative attitudes to be transmuted through the silver, gold, and pearlescent flames. One may need to spend more time in this flame to prepare properly for the transformation to come. Allow the violet flame to reinstate balance and wholeness and clear the path to freedom; with it, you will burn through the brush to see the clearing ahead.*

On the long drive from Colorado to Chicago, Peregrine and Alice—each seat-belted into the cab of a noisy U-Haul truck—alternated between chatting, singing with the radio, and daydreaming out the window. As they reached sight of Chicago's famous skyline, Peregrine was again ready for a new adventure: she had enrolled in a graduate program in Oriental medicine. She intended to take the many lessons she had learned in the Hebrides and in Colorado, and the whole of her life's journey, and expand on them as an actual career. This truly was a direct result of a conscious life change.

As they neared the city, Peregrine's heart beat faster with anticipation and empowerment. She had never been to Chicago before. She'd rented an apartment online after hours of research, including talking with a few people at the acupuncture school about neighborhoods near good school districts for Alice. In the end, she chose a neighborhood close to downtown that had a great school for Alice, as well as being close to all the perks the city had to offer. Peregrine was excited to move Alice to a city with all the opportunities for exploration, challenge, and self-expression she had so sorely craved as a child. Alice, now in first grade, smiled back at her from the passenger seat before glancing back out the window. Peregrine could tell by her rapt gaze that she was excited to see the city bustling. This was a complete juxtaposition to the serene, still landscape of the Colorado mountains.

Here, just as in Colorado—and Paris many years ago— Peregrine vowed to open up even further to being exactly who she was. Rather than *creating* a new persona, she saw it as an unlayering, the act of stripping herself bare to her truest core. People would love her for it or they wouldn't. Peregrine would be okay with either scenario.

Their apartment was just north of downtown, a short walk to Michigan Avenue. Four guys in coveralls waited in front of the row-house buildings; the screen-printed logo crossing their backs matched the ad Peregrine had picked for moving muscle, and they waved her into the loading zone in front of the building. An hour and a half later, Peregrine and Alice were settling in with all their belongings. Once again, the antique green velvet couch, Chinese tables, and other antiques found places in their new digs. Peregrine and, she suspected, Alice both wondered silently what was ahead of them.

As it turned out, Chicago was a friendly city, and Peregrine quickly met the other mothers at Alice's school; indeed, they all seemed to live within a five-block radius of the apartment. A lot of the mothers didn't work, so Peregrine found an instant neighborhood support group where Alice could have play dates if Peregrine needed to be at school. Alice made friends almost immediately, and Peregrine was grateful that, as calm and levelheaded as Alice was, she didn't seem to have inherited her mother's natural introversion. It was a quality Peregrine resolved to keep pulling away from in Chicago. She wanted to be as open as Alice was, letting go of the mistrust and protectiveness that shielded her true personality. Nothing appealed to her more, at this point in her life, than teaching herself to be comfortable enough with others—and in her own skin—to let her inner beauty shine. Alternative medicine grad school, with all its focus on wholeness, seemed the perfect place to do that.

Peregrine had planned her four years of graduate school carefully. She'd saved enough money to get by for two years without a job, cramming in as many classroom hours as possible while Alice was at school. When Alice returned to New Orleans to visit her father and grandparents for the summer, Peregrine would work as many clinic hours as she could. Her goal was to complete her classroom hours in two years, then get a part-time job to support herself and Alice as she finished her clinical requirements.

Peregrine enrolled in twenty-four credit hours—nearly a double load—that semester. It was a tough schedule, and Peregrine spent more time with her classmates than she did with Alice. It wasn't long before the other students started to feel like family.

Peregrine only got about three hours of solid sleep a night. Then she made breakfast for Alice and dropped her off at school before running along Lake Michigan. Some days, she clocked up to seven or eight miles. She'd learned to quiet her mind and meditate while running, which almost made up for the lost sleep—an immense benefit since a quick shower and then school came right after her run.

Alternative medicine school was often a harsh contrast between Western and Eastern medical philosophies. Anatomy, physiology, pharmacology, microbiology, and biochemistry were juxtaposed with Chinese Confucius and Taoist philosophy, herbalism, acupuncture point location, and Oriental medicine theory classes. Then there were needling practice sessions and psychological therapeutic classes. The Western medical courses trained students to look at the body as an engine, pulling it apart to examine the muscles, the tendons, the veins, the nerves; the body was a piece of material that could be manipulated and "fixed," just as Andrew used to restore antique cars. Then Peregrine walked into the Eastern medical classes, where suddenly the body was a unit of an eco-system, with cycles of life and an intrinsic connection to the mind and spirit. She learned about energy meridians that passed longitudinally through the body and how there were points on the soles of one's feet and the palms of one's hands that correlated and connected to every bodily structure. She learned how a person's liver had its own spirit residing within it, and how, when that spirit's energy became unbalanced, physical and psychological effects in other body systems occurred. Her brain was constantly switching between East and West, and she found, again and again, that the holistic approach felt like home. However, the two methods still had a space to meet in the middle.

One of the lessons Peregrine found most fascinating was the idea that everything had an energetic property and energetics could be manipulated. Of course, she knew the human body was an electrical system—even allopathic medicine had the system of neurology—but it made Peregrine place more importance on her own energy, what she was expelling into the world and to those around her. She realized that in order to *receive* clean, pure, positive energy from others, she needed to give the same. Meditation was a way to cultivate the calm, serene mind that would allow for that kind of energetic output.

In order to truly meditate, Peregrine used a visualization technique. At night, she lay on her back in bed, hands by her sides and legs in a straight line. She closed her eyes and imagined that the top of her head was connected to a plug in her headboard, which had a tube extending straight through the sky to never-ending infinity. From that place of mystery poured bright white light, strong and pure, and every time Peregrine inhaled, she visualized the white light flowing through the tube and the top of her head, all the way down to her toes. Then, on her exhale, the light streamed vertically out through her fingertips, her toes, her nose, and her eyelids, shooting back into the world. Peregrine visualized every capillary, every vein, every atom in her body completely replaced by white light. It was like completely cleansing her body before she went to sleep, and when Peregrine woke up, it was with intense clarity and energy.

Though her days and nights were full and invigorating, there were times Peregrine felt lonely. She missed the friends she'd made in Colorado, and she was entering such a state of self-acceptance and self-love that she wanted to share it with others. She decided the only way to build relationships was to invite them. Consciously, with intention, she put out positive energy through smiling and initiating conversations with students in her classes and with parents she met through Alice's school. That was how she met Brennan.

Brennan was a wealthy entrepreneur whose son was in Alice's class. They met at the kids' Christmas pageant. Peregrine was sitting in the middle of the auditorium when he walked in through a door by the stage. He was tall, with dark hair and eyes and an impeccable body. Immediately, despite the buzz of movement in the room, their eyes met. Peregrine froze, startled by the strong, instant connection that lingered in her spirit even after he'd disappeared from her peripheral vision. The next thing she knew, he was sitting beside her. She felt as though she were crawling out of her skin. He was an energy vampire, draining Peregrine even as he excited her. She instantly knew this wasn't going to be good, but she was willing to take the journey anyway.

"So, why haven't I seen you here before?" he asked, after they'd introduced themselves.

Peregrine smiled coyly. "Maybe you haven't looked in the right place."

"I see." His deep brown eyes lit with intrigue. "And where's Alice's dad tonight?"

"He's in New Orleans."

"Too bad for him." Brennan's eyes crinkled in the corners, and Peregrine took swift inventory of his own ringless finger. "Come out with me tonight, then," he said. "After the pageant."

"Just like that, huh?" Peregrine laughed, attracted to Brennan's confidence (or, more accurately, arrogance). It swept her back to her Paris exchange with Alexandre. The match was on.

"Just like that. I've got my sitter's number on speed dial."

"Father of the year."

Peregrine felt heady with their banter, and she couldn't help but notice the tender look that entered Brennan's eyes when he gazed at his son on stage. No man who looked at his child like that could be all that bad. She was both right and wrong.

Peregrine looked at him and smiled. "Just make it worth my time."

By the end of the night, Peregrine and Brennan were kissing passionately in the back of a cab, and her mind was working overtime trying to remember what under-wear she'd put on that morning. Though she had dated in Colorado, she hadn't been in a serious relationship in—how long—so underwear hadn't been an issue in a while. Not that she was considering Brennan "serious" potential. She was happy to enjoy the moment she was in for exactly what it was worth: fun, chemistry, and sheer physical pleasure. As with Alexandre, Peregrine felt powerful in her beauty and sexuality. She wanted to express it.

"Come to my place?" Brennan asked against her lips.

Peregrine nodded, her hands in his hair.

"One stop," he told the cab driver.

. . .

At twenty-nine, Peregrine was among the youngest in most of her courses. The students ranged from their thirties to their fifties and came from a wide variety of life paths: some had been Western medical doctors before changing careers; some owned yoga studios; some had traveled so extensively it made Peregrine's own globetrotting seem trivial. As the year progressed, Peregrine felt they were getting to know one another on a more intimate level than she'd ever experienced with classmates or colleagues. They were all required to divulge their physical and psychological health issues so they could practice therapeutic work on one another. They were trained to see through facades; if someone were not being completely honest and authentic, he or she would be called out on it. At first, this was scary to Peregrine. There was nowhere to hide! Then she realized, *No one could hide.* Without any choice, Peregrine was getting exactly what she wanted: these people were all going to know her for who she was, and she was going to know them. She couldn't control the situation, which was scary, but at least it was mutual. The challenge of transparency was exactly what she'd wanted upon coming to Chicago.

Still, Peregrine fought her familiar introversion. Though she was very close to the people in her class, she hardly spoke to anyone outside it. In clinic, where classes were mixed, there were days she arrived and left without speaking to anyone but the patients. One day, just as Peregrine was about to leave, she crossed paths with a woman in her class. She was blond, a little hippie, casually dressed in a t-shirt and jeans. Peregrine knew her name was Angela and that she was a yoga instructor, and she could tell from the way Angela spoke up in class that she was brassy and opinionated.

"Hey, what's up?" Angela asked casually.

"Nothing," Peregrine responded.

Angela waited a beat and then laughed. "That's it?"

"I guess so."

"You don't talk much, do you? What's the matter, not interested in making friends?"

Peregrine shrugged, blushing slightly. "I'm just in a rush. I don't mean to be rude."

Angela evaluated her for a moment, looking amused. "Hey, Hollywood Dan," she called back to the guy with whom she usually shared a table. "Guess what? She's not a bitch!"

Peregrine's eyes widened. "You thought I was a bitch?"

Angela laughed. "Don't take it personally. You're just so direct. You roll in here, grab and stab all the patients, and take off. We thought you were stuck up. I thought, 'Uh, uh, I have to go talk to this girl, I can't stand one more day on the sidelines.'"

Peregrine would have taken offense were it not for the laughter in Angela's voice. "Well, now you know." As an afterthought, she added with a grin, "Bitch."

"All right, that's it!" Angela said, grabbing Peregrine's hand. "Dan and I are getting drinks tonight. You're coming."

"Actually, I've got to make dinner for my daughter. But I'm in for tomorrow if you guys want."

"Consider it a date."

Two weeks after their first conversation, Peregrine and Angela were inseparable. They drank, sat on the beach, went to Cubs games, spent leisurely afternoons shopping on Michigan Avenue, or just lingered in the coffee shop for hours of conversation. "You are my female soulmate," Angela often said, and Peregrine—who had never thought such a thing was possible—wholeheartedly agreed. When she and Angela were together, there was no part of their personalities they didn't share. Peregrine told Angela everything about herself and her past; after a while, she came to think there was not one thing Angela did not know about her.

One aspect of their friendship that Peregrine both loved and loathed was that Angela never just told her what she wanted to hear. Good god, Peregrine wished she would sometimes, because the truth could be brutal. "That is the stupidest thing I have ever heard," Angela might say. Or, severely: "I expect more from you than that." Angela didn't let Peregrine get away with a stitch of dishonesty or deception, and she had no problem calling out her inconsistencies, fears, and doubts. Oddly, it built the most trusting relationship Peregrine had ever experienced—and paved the way for Peregrine to do the same for others—because she knew that no matter how harsh Angela was, she'd always be there to listen to the next thing. She never hung up the phone without saying, "I love you," despite whatever knock-down, drag-out fight they'd just had, and Peregrine knew that love was unconditional. It was new for her. Other than Mimi, she'd never had strong female influences in her life, and this was a friendship she knew she'd always treasure.

Still … she didn't particularly enjoy one of their recurring arguments—which was over Brennan. When the three of them spent time together, Angela didn't restrain the look of disgust at his arrogance or the way he shamelessly flirted with other women. Afterwards, she'd say to Peregrine, "I just hate that guy. I can't believe you sink down to his level."

Peregrine just responded, "He's not that bad. He's *such* a good father. And he's great to Alice. Besides, it's not like this is serious. We're just having fun."

But Peregrine's words fell flat, even to her own ears. The truth was, they *were* having fun. When they were together, their banter was pointed and witty. They were constantly touching—a stroke of the arm, a snuck kiss on a nape of the neck, a hand on the thigh—and flirting, and when they were in bed … it was all the openness and sensuality of Paris plus the self-confidence and maturity the years since had lent. When Peregrine was entangled in Brennan's arms and his dark eyes soaked the entirety of her in, she saw a chance for *more* in this relationship. And those moments were precisely when Brennan withdrew. An arm slid from beneath her, a lamp flicked off, and a casual, "I'm heading to LA tomorrow for two weeks. I'll give you a call when I get back," reminded Peregrine that his heart was unavailable. The intensity of their chemistry against the abruptness of his emotional departure was a strange dichotomy that kept Peregrine constantly uncertain.

"'Just having fun,'" Angela scoffed. "It doesn't matter, Peregrine. You deserve better than how he treats you. You know he's got to have a girl in every city he lands in for his 'business trips.'"

They glared at each other. Then Angela let out a huffing sigh and shook her head. "I just love you, girl."

"I know," Peregrine grumbled. "I love you, too."

In a way, these endings to their arguments reflected what Peregrine was learning in class. There, she was taught that to be a healer, she had to work on herself constantly. She had to be energetically clean and pure, coming from an egoless place in order not to interfere with somebody else's healing or energy.

"When working with patients, your path is not the point," the instructor related. "Their health is, and your only place is to help facilitate their wellness. That means putting aside your judgment. The patient's political, religious, and social positions do not matter. Someone has come to you for assistance and healing, and you will not be able to help them if you're not connected to pure, unlimited potential."

Unlimited potential . . . Peregrine pondered the phrase. More and more, she was recognizing that most actions are of the ego, formulated out of fear, misunderstanding, prejudices, and past hurts. When treating people, she needed to look at them through eyes of pure positive love, which she now saw was at the core of every human being. Most people were seeking to give and receive unconditional love and alignment for their true selves, through which an unlimited potential of expansion could bloom. She realized that to connect with other human beings on a level that would help guide them to a place of true love for themselves and a place of unlimited potential, she needed to lead by example. *She* needed to expand. She needed to look straight into the white light of someone's heart and let all the other facades melt away as wax from a candle.

Letting go of judgment—for herself as well as others—was immensely freeing. She'd been fearful that her classmates would find her weak or broken when she opened herself to tears and misgivings. Yet, each time she watched them be vulnerable and open, she saw bravery and strength. Every class, every interaction, seemed to open Peregrine up to new self-revelation and maturity. She recognized again that the events of her life—good and bad—were of her own choosing. She had to admit her accountability, her role in her actions. Peregrine was reminded of her stay in the Hebrides, the sense of interconnectedness she'd felt, and the liberation that came from owning her mistakes. She saw that compromising one's authentic self meant gaining fear and doubt, and losing unlimited potential and pure love. When Peregrine thought of pure love, she considered it first a love within herself, then like having a connection to something higher. It was one heart connecting to another through a pathway of white light with no strings attached.

Peregrine's realizations were a double-edged sword for her relationship with Brennan. She saw his potential so clearly, so brightly—he was brilliant and driven, a self-made millionaire who cared deeply about his business. Peregrine often woke up to find him tapping quietly on his laptop in the living room at three in the morning. He'd look up in the glow with eyes far too alert for that hour and smile at her. "I'm just wrapping up. I'll look in on David and be there in a few minutes." Peregrine would smile back, kiss him, and tread sleepily back to a bed that would remain empty for the rest of the night. Brennan's drive inspired

Peregrine to do more in her life. She was fully committed to school, giving all of herself to learning how to heal, but what about after that? Her old dream of being a doctor was gone; what was rising up in its place? Brennan helped inspire these thoughts, and she was starting to look to him as a model for making something out of nothing. In many ways, he lived the life he'd always dreamed of. It made her think the same was possible for her.

What Peregrine loved most about Brennan, though, was the kind of father he was. No matter how busy, he made it to David's parent/teacher conferences, his science fairs, his Little League games. He made him dinner and tucked him in at night. He read him stories and hugged and kissed him with none of the reserve some men possessed for showing their sons affection. And he treated Alice as his own. He was warm and loving and attentive, and when Peregrine watched him helping Alice with her homework, she could imagine a future with him ... if only there wasn't something so important missing.

Brennan's first marriage had ended with his wife's affair, followed by her taking half his money. The glimpses of openness Peregrine saw in him—the ones that kept her in the relationship—were immediately followed by a cool shutting of doors that could only mean one thing: Brennan was guarding his love, and that made Peregrine keep hers at bay as well. That wasn't the relationship she wanted. She wanted someone who was willing to journey with her, to expand to their highest potential together. In her gut, she knew Brennan wasn't that man. She understood she was walking down the path of old mistakes.

On her evening runs, Peregrine asked herself what she needed to do in her personal life to cultivate the greatest expansion of her unlimited potential. What could she be doing to clean up her past mistakes, old judgments, and old disserving habits in order to manifest her dreams? She could have anything she wanted . . . if only she knew clearly what that was and what was preventing her from seeing it.

"It seems like so long ago that I was married to Andrew, miserable with my life," Peregrine mused one night to Angela. They were sitting at their favorite bar, rounding out their second gin and tonic. She shuddered. "I almost can't believe that was me."

"Well, it was," Angela said simply. "A you that was learning, just like you're still learning."

Angela's matter-of-factness struck Peregrine as profound. Often over the years, she'd tried to disassociate from her past; she'd forgiven herself, moved on, and that was it. But she realized now that in that disengagement, there was judgment. She was not showing herself all the love and acceptance she deserved.

"I am still learning," Peregrine said thoughtfully. She lifted her glass to her lips but didn't take a sip. "I'm writing a new story. I can't keep ending it the same way."

"What are you talking about?" Angela asked.

Peregrine met her best friend's eyes. "Brennan."

Angela sighed. "I'm sorry that I am so hard on you about that. You know I will support whatever you think is best for you. Just make it the best."

Peregrine nodded. Her chest felt tight with the decision she was making, but she knew it was the right one. To be true to herself, she could not accept a relationship with someone who wasn't a true match. As much good as there was in the relationship, as much potential as Brennan possessed, it simply wasn't completely fulfilling to her. She needed to be inspired to expand in all directions, and she knew she would be settling again if she stayed with him. This was a decision of real self-love—to let something go in order to make room for the relationship that had *real* unlimited potential. She deserved that kind of beauty in her life … and that was exactly what she was going to manifest.

Debrief

DISTILLATION: VIOLET FLAME

The violet flame is the "mother of the stone." It is the connection between mind and body, softening our karma and allowing us to learn from past mistakes. It prepares us to ascend to the higher flames by raising our vibration closer to JOY, readying us for manifesting our true beauty. It accomplishes this by transmuting our negative, limiting beliefs into positive energy in order to realize our unlimited potential as human beings. It can purify past traumas, cleanse and soften our karma, and inspire us to seek out our destiny. The violet flame can restore energy back to its original state of purity, cleansing our karmic vibrations not by erasing, but by shifting negative energy to positive. What are your negative thought patterns that need to be changed? ☙ What are your blockages? ☙ Your old habits? ☙ Old patterns? ☙ Where do you need to shift your energy? ☙ In forgiving your past mistakes or others' past mistakes, have you let go of the judgments, too? ☙ What needs to heal in your life for your unlimited potential to be realized? ☙ Take inventory of the situations in your life to see if there are areas where you are settling. Could they be greater? ☙ What is the new story you would like to write?

CHAPTER 7

Silver Flame

SILVER FLAME: *The silver flame is the sister flame to the gold flame. It is the moon to the gold's sun. Its hallmarks are femininity and love, energy that allows you to treat issues of separation, illusion, and self-doubt. This is the time to discover your truest desires, to explore your feminine strength and energy, and to dream up your beautiful intentions.*

*I*n Peregrine's last year of acupuncture school, she worked full time in a perfume company. Her main task was to handle accounts payable, but the environment returned her to a lifelong love of creating scents. She balanced her passion for perfume making by capitalizing on daily opportunities to learn about manufacturing and product development, packaging, and branding. Meanwhile, her evening job at the acupuncture school's clinic gave her endless opportunities to put the theory she'd learned in classes to the test of actual human experience.

After a busy July day at work, Peregrine mentally and physically shifted gears as she headed to her shift in the clinic. She traded her business suit jacket for a lab coat, washed the faded makeup from her face, and reapplied a minimal look, purposefully changing personas as she changed her uniform. Concentrating on her breath, she strove to connect to *this* space and time, exhaling the remaining busy-ness of her office environment and inhaling white light and the healing space around her. Peregrine strode into the clinic hoping that she'd sufficiently made the transition for the good of all.

Tonight she was on the middle floor of the three-level facility, each holding about twenty-five beds, curtained off as one might expect in an emergency room. Sitting on the rolling exam stool by the bed, she observed her first patient, a middle-aged, somewhat overweight woman. She glanced at the woman's intake form, which indicated she was experiencing back pain.

The woman, whose name was Joan, wrapped one hand around her lower back. "I clean offices every night, so I'm headed to work shortly, but aspirin isn't cutting it anymore."

Peregrine explained that external physical pain was often a manifestation of an internal ailment. Although she seemed slightly doubtful about the process, Joan patiently answered all of Peregrine's questions about her eating habits, her digestion, exercise, migraines, work environment, and family history—not just of back pain, but other sorts of diseases and emotional traumas. She followed Peregrine's instructions to stand up, walk about twenty feet down the aisle, then turn and walk back to her bed. Peregrine watched her gait closely. Afterwards, she took Joan's pulse and made note not only of its rate, but also how strong it felt and how easy it was to find in her wrist. She asked if she could examine Joan's tongue and noted whether it was coated or clear, shaky or calm, swollen or normal looking.

She asked a series of questions about the qualities of Joan's back pain—whether it felt sharp and stabbing or dull and achy, what times of the day it intensified, whether it was worse in the heat of summer or the cold of winter, when she bent over or stood still.

Over the nearly thirty-minute interview, Peregrine became clearer and clearer on which meridians were most strongly connected to Joan's health and, specifically, to her back pain. She asked Joan to remove her blouse and put on a gown with the opening facing the back. "I'll be back in a few to give you your treatment."

Joan's face grew a bit taut. "Will it hurt?" she asked, voicing the question Peregrine knew had been on her mind the whole time.

"No," Peregrine said with a smile. "Don't worry; you won't feel like a pincushion."

Peregrine stepped away from the partitioned area, closed her eyes, and sought to release fully the stresses of her day and week. Try as she might, though, she still felt off-centered and distracted. The white light trick wasn't working as well for her today. She must be tired. Pushing past her feelings, she stepped through the curtain to her patient again. But as she inserted the first needle, Joan yelped in pain.

"I'm so sorry!" Peregrine said.

Damn it, she thought. She recognized, once again, the enormous difference it made when she wasn't fully centered before touching a patient. She pulled the needle and placed one gloved hand on Joan's back in what she intended as a calming gesture. She put the other gloved hand on the edge of the table. With the intention of connecting with grounding earth energy, she closed her eyes momentarily, exhaled deeply, and then inhaled. *Exhale dark and gray negativity, inhale beauty and light, pure energy, and healing.* This time, she could feel it work as her hands tingled.

"Let's try this again," Peregrine said calmly.

Joan's back was tense, but Peregrine applied some healing massage to the area before carefully inserting another needle. This time, however, she made no noise at all, nor did she move or make a sound as Peregrine efficiently placed fifteen more needles along her spine. Soon, Joan fell into the deep relaxation that Peregrine had come to expect in all her patients. Peregrine spent the next thirty minutes repeating the intake process with another patient. When she returned to remove the needles, Joan looked at her with a face so relaxed she looked like a different person. That was more like it, she thought.

. . .

Finally back home at eleven p.m., Peregrine checked her voicemail and email for messages from Alice, who was staying with Mimi this week, and then made herself a big fresh salad for her late-night dinner. After eating, she sat down in her dining room for what she considered her third job.

Her dining room was a makeshift lab, where Peregrine was combining the healing components of her studies with the beauty of perfume. In a heady rush, she remembered Mimi's Shalimar, the Paris tours of perfumeries large and small, and the signature scent she'd worn until its last drop. Here, late at night at her table, she conducted her own research and development, blending different therapeutic essential oils for aromatherapy. The hours passed quickly as Peregrine lost herself in concentration and the distinctly feminine energy of her work. She felt softer in the presence of her perfumes—more sensual, nurturing, and dreamy. There was a calm here that she didn't feel very often, a space where she could breathe and allow herself to be Peregrine the *woman*—not Peregrine the head of the household or Peregrine the accounts payable manager or Peregrine the hardworking student. It was such a refreshing, renewing feeling that she didn't realize the time until it was two a.m. With a tender sigh, she cleaned her "lab" area and padded to her bedroom for a few hours of sleep before starting the cycle again tomorrow.

The next day was Friday, and Angela called her after clinic with a purpose: "You *have* to come out! Come dance with me! Then tomorrow we'll head north to Madison and hang at my family's farm there for the rest of the weekend. You need a break even worse than I do, girl!"

So they danced themselves almost into oblivion. Then, promising never to drink another drop of alcohol, they drove to Madison the next morning for a quieter sort of relaxation. By the time they reached their favorite restaurant, they broke their promise, ordering mimosas with brunch.

"Cheers to the hair of the dog," Angela toasted. But today, at least, they each stopped at just one glass. By midday, they were sipping club soda with twists of lime, stretched out side by side on chaise lounges on the back deck, soaking up the sunshine.

Angela sighed in contentment. "Do you know that the largest Tibetan Buddhist monastery in the whole Western world is just twenty minutes from here?"

Peregrine sat up straight. "Get out! Why are you just telling me this now? We've been to Madison how many times?"

"I don't know. I mean—"

"Why aren't we there now?"

"Didn't think you'd latch onto that so quickly!" Angela said, laughing. "We'll go tomorrow."

The next morning, Angela parked the car in front of Deer Park Buddhist Center, and a Tibetan monk came out to meet them. Bowing slightly, his hands pressed together over his heart, he said, "Welcome to Deer Park. My name is Anil."

Peregrine almost gasped aloud. He was beautiful—six foot two or so, with a smooth cinnamon skin and serene brown eyes. She glanced at Angela, biting back a giggle. How wrong was it that she found the monk to be quite sexy? But Angela's own attention was on the building beyond Anil. The architecture was remarkable, unlike anything Peregrine had seen in the States or Europe. A roof with corners that curled towards the sky; gorgeous red, gold, and blue intricate painted designs along the entryway; two deer sculptures flanking a teardrop-shaped emblem at the top of the roof—the place was clearly designed as a temple from another culture.

"Would you like a tour, or would you prefer to wander on your own?" Anil asked.

"We'll do the tour, thanks," Peregrine said quickly, with her own agenda in mind. She avoided Angela's knowing gaze.

They followed Anil across the manicured lawns. His stride was smooth and graceful, and his commentary mostly focused on the architecture rather than on Buddhism. He often showed them something, said a few words, and then sat with eyes closed, allowing them to do the same.

Peregrine and Angela started out chatty but found themselves drawn to follow Anil's lead. Soon, Peregrine was paying as much or more attention to the birds singing in the trees, the sound of the limbs and branches shifting in the breeze, and the sensation of sunshine on her bare arms. The peacefulness was profound.

From the temple, they heard a gong chime once. "We have about half an hour before formal meditation begins," Anil said. "If you'd like, I can show you the public spaces within the temple before the ceremony."

"Let's do it," Angela said, and off they went, down the hill toward the temple. Inside was an abundance of color and gold leaf and Buddha imagery.

"What's upstairs?" Peregrine asked after they seemed to have toured the entire main floor.

"There are a number of apartments for the Rinpoche and other monks and, of course, a special one reserved for the Dalai Lama when he visits."

"The Dalai LAMA!" Angela and Peregrine said in unison.

"Please," Peregrine said. "You have to show it to us."

"It's not as luxurious as you might think," he said, "and it's really not part of the public tour."

"We're only here for the day," Peregrine said beseechingly. "We won't be in anyone's way. He's not here today, right, and so it won't do any harm. Please?"

Somehow, Anil relented and took them up a hidden stairway. Angela winked at Peregrine and whispered, "Flirting with a monk, now, Peregrine? Is this what you've come to?"

Peregrine grinned back. She was in the mood to start getting what she wanted!

At the top of the stairs, they rounded a corner and Anil glanced both ways down the hall before opening the door to the apartment and ushering them inside. They saw a small table with two chairs, a small loveseat and side chair, and a cabinet of Tibetan design against one wall. Through the doorway, they saw a bedroom with one twin bed, a nightstand, and dresser. The furniture was sparse but ornate— a beautiful combination of serene simplicity and intense beauty. The mix was awe inspiring.

"He likes to say, 'I am a simple monk,'" Anil said. "And this is his preference."

At the sound of another chime, Anil said, "The meditation will begin shortly, and I will be needed downstairs."

Peregrine and Angela followed Anil to the main room of the temple. The large, square area felt airy beneath a soaring twenty-foot ceiling, with an altar at the back that seemed to glow supernaturally blue. Centered was a fifteen-foot tall golden Buddha statue, with a number of other Buddha representations on shelves around it. In front, people sat in quiet meditation on rows of flat, square cushions. The monks moved fluidly in their robes, finding their own positions of prayer, and though no one was speaking, there was a communal vibration of joy that stirred Peregrine and Angela to silence.

After a few minutes, a noise at Peregrine's elbow startled her, and she turned to see Angela with tears streaming down both cheeks.

Angela took a shuddering breath. "It's so beautiful, Peregrine," she whispered.

Peregrine smiled and reached for Angela's hand. She held it silently, sharing in her friend's emotional moment. They stood that way, appreciating the beautiful energy of the space around them, until Angela took another deep breath and nodded. Peregrine nodded back, warm with gratitude to have shared this day with Angela.

Outside, a fresh cool breeze washed over them both, and the bright sunlight nearly blinded them. Once they reached the bottom of the steps, Angela said, "Let's sit outside a few minutes before we go back."

To Peregrine's surprise, Anil's soft voice called from behind them. "There is one thing you haven't seen."

Peregrine and Angela turned. "Don't they need you in the temple?"

"I will take a moment to show you."

Soon they were walking with Anil back across the lawn to a monument that looked rather like a large white chess piece, sort of a cross between a pawn and a bishop. "This is our stupa, a place for quiet meditation. You see the form? It represents a sitting Buddha. The Dalai Lama came here to dedicate it at the time of the Kalachakra Initiation."

A series of tall poles surrounded the stupa, with lines connecting them in gentle curves. Along each line and every possible way to connect two high points, strings of Tibetan prayer flags were hung. Each flag in each series—blue, white, red, green, yellow—had images of windhorses (a Tibetan Buddhist allegory for the human soul) and strings of words written in a language indecipherable to Peregrine. There must have been hundreds of flags, some tattered and faded, many bright with color.

"People hang the flags here and release their prayers in the wind so goodwill and compassion go everywhere the wind blows," Anil said. "Listen." He closed his eyes and became silent. The sound of the flags waving and snapping seemed almost deafening at first, and then somehow shifted into a pleasant, simple, white-noise sound, comforting like the sound of clean laundry drying on a line outside. Even with the flags, Peregrine could hear birdsong, undeterred by the prayer flags' own melody.

Without words, Peregrine and Angela each found one of the single-seat marble benches and sat facing the sun, eyes closed, quiet. For once, Peregrine's mind really did seem to stop chattering, leaving her only with sensation: breeze, bench, scent, sunlight glowing through closed eyelids. And a new voice inside her head: *Just listen.*

So she did. Many wordless insights came to her at once, just knowing, not thinking. *Every thought you think is a choice, and through those thoughts, you create reality.*

Any feeling other than happiness is merely a sign that you've allowed something to go wrong; for the moment, you're not in alignment with your true nature. The feeling is a signal, not a reality of its own, and it will pass once you realign yourself.

Your biggest gift is creating your own reality in the present moment.

The last thought—or "knowing"—made Peregrine shiver with a silvery sense of empowerment. She envisioned a beautiful store, luxurious tones of merlot and gold, filled with sparkling bottles of perfume that did more than smell good; they healed. The image in her mind was so vivid it was like a memory, as though she'd been there before. Then Peregrine realized it was more than a memory. It was the creation of reality, born right in the peaceful, feminine energy of this moment.

Peregrine opened her eyes and smiled at Angela, whose face was open and peaceful.

"Let's get on the road," Peregrine said. "I have a lot to do when we get home."

Debrief

COAGULATION: SILVER FLAME

The silver flame is the feminine counterpart to the gold flame; one cannot exist without the other. As the moon illuminates the water on a lake, the silver flame casts gentle light on your deepest desires. It embodies the feminine dreamer energy and sets the stage for the gold flame to bring forth the riches of what your mind has created. Look at your life's desires, passions, and joy to envision all of what can and shall be. Use everything you have learned from the lower flames to create an everlasting story of a beautiful life. The silver flame is your crystal ball, and you are the creator of your future. The gold flame will help you manifest it into reality.

Rewrite your story. What are the deepest desires you want manifested? ❧ Have you looked into yourself under the still moonlight? ❧ What was hidden there? ❧ Are you ready to bring that forth and live your beauty?

CHAPTER 8

Gold Flame: Chicago

GOLD FLAME: *The gold flame brings about the masculine, assertive energy needed for true manifestation of dreams. The husband to the quiet silver flame, the gold flame provides the vision to see opportunities and the energy to sustain the motivation behind the desires.*

Peregrine had finished her acupuncture training, and a couple weeks later, she and Alice visited her parents for Christmas. Over dessert, Peregrine made their announcement: they were staying in Chicago until Alice finished the school year in May, and then they would move back to New Orleans—for the long term—the next summer. Peregrine wanted Alice to spend her high school years near her father and extended family. She was dreading the return home but tried to think of it as an opportunity: if she could take back with her all the lessons she'd learned, maybe she could conquer the place that had stifled her all her life. In the meantime, she would continue her full-time job in the perfume store while setting the foundation for achieving her true desire: opening her own perfumery so she could combine her passion fragrance with the healing tools she'd learned in acupuncture school. Now more than ever,

Peregrine felt the path toward the beautiful life she wanted before her; the weeds were gone, and her only task was daring to walk the very road she'd worked so hard to clear.

Peregrine's father gazed at her with tenderness in his eyes. "You know what you want," he said. "Go after it."

Mimi was rosy with pleasure at Peregrine's confidence and conviction. "*That's* my girl," she said, squeezing Peregrine's hand and smiling across the table at Alice. "I am so proud of you for finding who you are and living the life you want."

Even Peregrine's mother couldn't object to her plan. Anyone who looked at Peregrine could see that she was a woman on a mission—determined, passionate, and radiating the energy that comes at the cusp of fulfillment.

Back in Chicago, Peregrine suddenly had time in what felt like luxurious amounts compared to her previous schedule. Each weekday, she left her job promptly at five. She grabbed the train and arrived home just as Alice returned from her extracurricular activities at school. The two of them chatted and prepared dinner together, and then Alice went to her room to finish her homework while Peregrine sat down to work on her aromatherapy and perfume blends. She loved working in both mediums, because the aromatherapy blends possessed healing tools, while the perfumes told stories. Together, they infused Peregrine with the joy of creating something truly beautiful.

She always started her work sessions by reviewing her notes on blends she'd created in the previous weeks. Peregrine kept a detailed notebook that included dates and specifications for each blend: what quantity of the inert foundation oil, how many drops of what particular base note scent, the number of drops of the middle note and the top note. Peregrine sterilized her kitchen counters and then covered them with fresh wax paper. Her bottles of essential oils, stored in light-tight boxes, were stretched out in a row and organized by type.

Two or three weeks after an initial blend was made, Peregrine would open the blue glass bottle in which it was stored, use an eyedropper to place one drop on a paper smelling strip, and explore how the scent had changed over time. Sometimes unexpected things happened and tertiary scents appeared, and sometimes the balance shifted and Peregrine would add a few more drops of the scent that had drifted away, always carefully adding the information to her notebook for future reference. She never knew when she might hit upon success and need to replicate it.

One night, in fact, Peregrine had started working with the perfume formula that she'd made years ago during her visit to Paris but decided to adapt it to reflect the depth in her life she'd acquired since then. In the original perfume, one whiff transported her to that amazing first night she'd had with Alexandre: the leather interior of his car, the spices in the dinner they ate together, and a faint wisp of his own musky cologne. The scent oozed of sensuality in complex, wondrous ways. Now she wanted the top notes to replicate her previous blend, to give her that familiar boost from the original experience, so her sense memory would help her step into the bold self she'd revealed that night in that amazing red silk gown. She kept the middle notes of her previous blend, too, to help her recollect her favorite memories of wearing her trademark scent during her first months and years back in New Orleans. But she wanted to adapt the base notes to reflect the complexity of her life today: she wasn't nineteen anymore, and she wanted to celebrate all she'd gained since then.

Around midnight, Peregrine's cell phone beeped. It was Angela, who must be getting off her clinic hours. *Can I stop in?*

Always. Text me and I'll buzz you in. Don't ring bell.

Half an hour later, Angela arrived with a bottle of wine and a wide grin. "I figured out the missing piece to our idea," she said, referring to the business concept she and Peregrine had been inventing together. They'd talked about one day presenting seminars or holding some sort of retreats, but they didn't feel they had the model quite right yet.

"All these women come to coaches, often struggling against some emotion—something they feel is holding them back. So we help them identify that emotion and understand why they're feeling it. 'Here's the Chinese medicine perspective, here's the *yoga perspective*, and here are some ways you can change it,'" Angela said, counting off the steps on her fingertips. "The yoga piece is what we were missing—the physical movement in addition to the philosophy."

Peregrine nodded, deep in the vision of their idea. "That's perfect," she said. "We don't want them just sitting there, with us doing all the talking. If we get them moving, they'll absorb and integrate the ideas much better. And it will bring breath and presence to their bodies in order to better identify, examine, and release the emotion—therefore addressing the problem in a more comprehensive way."

"Mind, body, and spirit," Angela agreed.

During their clinic work, both Peregrine and Angela had realized that so many people needed help organizing their lives, dealing with their stress, and raising their self-esteem, and acupuncture was only one tool to do that.

"Let's go with this some more," Angela said, pulling out her well-worn notebook for the project. "How would you get a client from here to there? From being stuck in the past to moving toward the future?"

"Let's ask them about their goals. 'It doesn't matter where you've been—where do you want to be, and where are you right now?' That's the key. We have to get them to acknowledge the very solid, honest truth about where they are *right now.* It doesn't mean they have to judge it—just acknowledge it."

Angela nodded as she wrote, and for a few minutes, they were both quiet and contemplative.

"Speaking of right now," Peregrine said, "let me share what I've been working on tonight." She rose to pull one of the little blue glass bottles from its lightproof box. She used the eyedropper to place one drop on Angela's left wrist.

Angela breathed deeply, eyebrows lifting in appreciation. "Ooh," she said. She closed her eyes and breathed in again. "It reminds me of driving fast in college, dark nights, and . . ." she grinned, "making out in the backseat of my boyfriend's car!"

Peregrine smiled back. "There's always a story behind perfume. Perfumers don't make scents that don't have stories. That said, though, perfumers might create a story that you *relate* to, but you make it your own as your body chemistry rewrites it."

"Perfume as storyteller," Angela mused. She breathed in again, smiling. "I like it."

Peregrine sighed. "It's not quite where I want it yet, but almost. I don't have the fixative right yet. I'm losing the top note already, and perfume should always be layered." Peregrine smiled, thinking of the vampire movies she used to watch with Mimi. "There's always more to it than meets the eye."

Angela ignored the obvious opportunity for a pun—*or the nose*—and instead told Peregrine firmly, "If anyone can get it right, you can."

After Angela left, Peregrine poured a glass of wine and sat alone with her thoughts. There was something about what she and Angela had been discussing—the potential of all the tools available to help people explore their current situation, goals, and desires. What if there was some way to incorporate just that into perfume making?

The moment the idea occurred to her, it was as though it had been there all along. This was it—the final piece. Peregrine jumped up from her chair, too excited to sit, and paced the living room floor. She remembered the vision of the perfume store she'd had at Deer Park and recalled the hundreds of times she'd sat with patients at clinic, asking them their stories in order to heal them. What if she could capture people's stories—past, present, and future—in a customized perfume, one smell of which would comfort, console, provoke, inspire, and ignite them into their true desires?

. . .

As the months passed, Peregrine continued to work at the perfume company and labored even harder each night at her kitchen table. She created perfume blends and aromatherapy mixtures, taking precise notes and thinking carefully about the stories she was telling through the scents—and for whom. The more people found out about Peregrine's work, the more she started receiving requests for customized blends. She created scents for everyone from Alice's friends' mothers—a specific aromatherapy blend of frankincense, myrrh, and lavender, for example, to rub over the stomach during menstruation—to friends and distant connections through acupuncture school. Her dining area was becoming more than a lab—it was becoming a manufacturing plant. Amber bottles, pipettes, glass stirrers, funnels, essential oil bottles, perfumers' alcohol, beeswax, label makers, wax paper, tin boxes for solid perfumes, and many scribbled notebooks covered the table, chairs, and countertops. Meanwhile, she was scouting online for locations in New Orleans that suited her beautiful vision of what this special perfumery would be. One by one, the pieces were clicking into place, and Peregrine's focus and resolve only grew as the days lengthened.

She did find herself, though, wanting to spend even more time with Angela than she'd anticipated before leaving. Over the last several years, their friendship had grown into a sisterhood that they both treasured.

"I've never seen you so sentimental!" Angela teased. They'd gone down to Mahoney's for drinks, as they had many a Friday night, especially while Alice was in New Orleans for the summer.

In their usual playful banter, Peregrine rolled her eyes. "Before you get too looped and your senses dull entirely, here, have this." She slid a small, wrapped box across the table toward Angela.

"A going-away present? But you're the one going away, not me," Angela said as she unwrapped the box. Looking at Peregrine with more kindness than her words belied, she continued, "You're not getting rid of me that easily. Whether my husband knows it or not, we'll be vacationing in New Orleans later this summer . . . and again in winter . . . and the spring . . ."

Inside the box was a lovely antique perfume bottle with a gold mesh atomizer bulb attached. Angela sighed softly, running her fingers over the bottle and holding it up to catch the prisms of light. "Just the bottle," she murmured. "It's beautiful. Is this one of yours?"

Peregrine smiled and nodded, feeling uncharacteristically jittery with anticipation.

Angela pumped a bit onto her wrist. When she lifted it to smell her nose, she closed her eyes and her face transformed. "Oh, Peregrine. I feel . . . transported." She looked at Peregrine with wonder. "It reminds of . . ." She breathed deeply again, " . . . that trip I told you about—the one to Arizona and New Mexico. How did you *do* that?"

Peregrine smiled, filled with pleasure and pride that her friend loved her customized scent. Long ago, Angela had told her about a trip she and her husband took and how they felt so connected with each other and with the earth. In the privacy of the empty desert, they were intimate and relaxed, utterly themselves and entirely united. With notes of piñon pine, purple sage, midnight cereus, and desert jasmine, the perfume smelled like the silence of open air, the cleanness of sparse vegetation, and the sensuality of the earth. "Oh, you know," Peregrine said, trying to shrug it off.

Angela sniffed her wrist again. "No, seriously. It's time to start selling this stuff instead of giving it away. You're going to make a fortune with this! This is your calling, girl."

"You know what?" Peregrine said, smiling. "I think so, too."

Debrief

MULTIPLICATION: GOLD FLAME

If the silver flame is as still as the moon on an evening lake, the gold flame is the sun beating down on a busy New York City sidewalk. This is where dreams are made! You have made your desires known and the gold flame engulfs them, feeds them, and pushes them out to the world. The gold flame is the masculine fire behind the feminine water of the silver flame, and they are harmonious together. In working with the gold and silver flames, you are connected to your higher self. You are self-aware and using energies from the previous flames to create and implement the beauty you seek in your life. The wealth of the gold flame will supply you with all the energy needed to implement your dreams and desires. You owe this to the world; inspire others to live out their beauty. The more oxygen you breathe into your gold flame, the brighter the world will be. The world needs more beauty.

What did you discover about your dreams and desires in the cool light of the silver flame? ᕙᕗ What resources do you need to implement your desires? ᕙᕗ How can you stay connected to your higher self in your course of action? ᕙᕗ Are you acting out of passion, desire, and authenticity? ᕙᕗ How can you best use your gold flame to actualize the beauty you have always dreamed of in your life?

CHAPTER 9

Pearlescent Flame: New Orleans

PEARLESCENT FLAME: *You hold the possibility of change based on your angle of illumination! The pearlescent flame is iridescent, from the Greek word iris, meaning "rainbow." Within a rainbow exists all color, all hope, all love, and all possibilities. Like a rainbow, the pearlescent flame holds the opportunity for all colors to shimmer on a surface as the angle of illumination changes. You, too, are iridescent.*

As Peregrine and Alice packed for their return to New Orleans, Peregrine's self-administered pep-talks were endless: this wasn't an ending but a beginning; not a concession but a challenge; not a return to an unhappy previous life but an opportunity to create the beautiful one she desired. As she filled boxes with treasures collected from her travels and oversaw her furniture being loaded into a moving van, she focused on both pouring out and soaking in positive energy. She took pleasure in the summer sun on her skin as she and Alice went for a last walk along Lake Michigan and took notice of how the water gently rippled with the motion of passing kayaks. Those ripples, she was certain, extended far beyond what she could see. Though they were leaving Chicago, the effects of their time here—and everywhere outside of New Orleans—would last as long Peregrine kept them close to her heart.

It took Peregrine and Alice a weekend to unpack and arrange their belongings in the small, but beautiful, antebellum home Peregrine had rented. Located in the Garden District, the home was all graceful wrought iron and cobblestone outside, on a street lined with ancient towering trees. Inside, floor to ceiling windows brightened the spaces she used as a home office and perfume lab, which she called the "perfumador." Sunlight gleamed off her grandmother's antiques and refracted on the more modern pieces Peregrine had integrated into the home. The overall effect was of a home with a story—a home perfect for a family.

Still, as Peregrine had suspected, readjusting to life in her hometown was far from easy. The muggy summer air coated her skin and frizzed her hair in a way that recalled her high school years of trying to fit in—trying *not* to make the water ripple—when she struggled with being different. Each day was a new challenge, an opportunity for her to practice reserving judgment, offering openness to connect to others, and upholding her authentic self. Over the years she had been gone, she'd built a completely new belief system about herself and the world, in addition to a career dramatically different from when she had dreamed of medical school. She'd turned her life into a work of art that was far beyond her younger imaginings. On days she was hard on herself for being negative about being back home, she reminded herself that she—like everyone—was still a work in progress, although she was much closer to a finished piece than those early brushstrokes.

"You've done a lot of work," Angela reminded her over the phone, "but you don't 'graduate' from life. You just have a new set of tools to work with and a much greater ability to recognize what tool is needed at any given point."

Peregrine nodded, pacing the floor of her bedroom. "I know . . . I think," she replied. "My beliefs and attitude about this place can be a heavy obstacle. I can't run away from it, and I can't ignore it. I don't want to fight it all the time, either."

"You said it yourself before you left—you are going to face your greatest challenge: to live in a previously suppressive place in total alignment with who you really are, which is your idea of complete freedom." Angela paused, and Peregrine could imagine her friend taking a sip of wine. They'd bought the same bottle for their phone date to recreate the experience of lounging on each other's couches in Chicago. "You know, it reminds me of that new perfume you sent me—doesn't it have pearl powder in it?"

"Yes," Peregrine said, smiling. Even the mention of perfume brought her calmness and peace. "It's for calming the spirit and soothing the emotions."

"Well, *you* know that for an oyster to make a pearl, it starts with a bit of an irritant—which is then transformed into a thing of beauty. That's what you're doing," Angela said. "Use your tools to transform this irritant into something beautiful and wondrous."

Peregrine, always one to retort with a witty one-liner rather than admit something had emotionally resonated, took a second to just breathe. "I like it," she said. "My job is to create the nacre."

"The what?" Angela laughed.

"The shiny outer coating of the pearl. Oysters use spit for the job—I guess I'm stuck with positivity as my tool."

The next morning, Peregrine arose feeling rejuvenated after her talk with Angela. She was ready to polish her tools and get to work making her pearl.

Peregrine found a job at one of the oldest perfumeries in the French Quarter. Though she eventually wanted to own her own business, she knew she needed steady income to support herself and Alice. Plus, this would be another training ground, a place where she could combine the complex intakes she'd learned in acupuncture school with the art of perfumery she so loved. Her idea was to customize blends for people using the knowledge she'd acquired about healing. Like a magical potion, perfume held the power to transform the emotional reality of the wearer, a subtle persuasion to change her physical reality. It could heal perceived damages and deficiencies in one's life and conjure the mystery and adventure of the future—or bring forth the memories of past joy and confidence. A perfume was never just a perfume. That was the attitude Peregrine took to work, and it was why she was developing a little following for her custom blends.

The perfumery drew foot traffic not only from tourists to the Quarter, but also from local women who came down to have their hair done at the elite salon and spa around the corner. When not busy making custom blends, Peregrine's days were usually spent replenishing stock, as a number of women purchased small samples of different perfumes and returned later for larger purchases of their favorites.

"My friend sent me here to speak with Miss Peregrine," said a woman in her early sixties as she entered the shop. She was beautiful and elegant with a long, swanlike neck adorned in a pearl necklace. Peregrine could easily see she had a classy, vain streak and the sort of comfortable lifestyle that afforded her that luxury.

"That's me," Peregrine said, tucking her gloves into the pocket of the custom designed jacket she always wore in the shop. "What can I do for you?"

"My name is Katheryn. My friend Grace, who always smells so lovely, told me you have created a perfume for her. I want to . . ." She looked around, a bit stealthily. "I want you to make a scent for me that you won't sell to anyone else," she said, one eyebrow arched.

Peregrine smiled. Her intuition was already providing a mental picture of the woman's dreams. "Of course. Have a seat here, and let's have a chat."

As Katheryn chattered about the events at which she intended to wear the new perfume, Peregrine observed how the woman structured her language about herself, the sto-ries she told—even the quality of her voice all unknowingly told tales of her wishes. Definitely, this was going to be a job for *perfume*! If Peregrine were creating aromatherapy, she'd need to come up with a blend of therapeutic scents that addressed someone's deficiencies and excesses according to the system of healing in which she was trained. However, when creating a perfume, she started with the therapeutics and then explored what the customer yearned to experience.

Often it was a memory, an emotion, a dream, or a journey. Based on that information, Peregrine explored what notes and scents, could conjure those feelings. Her goal was to invite customers into a world of olfactory transmutation that would take them where they wanted to go. And this woman definitely knew where she wanted to go.

After their half-hour conversation, Peregrine was left with one line that told her everything she needed to know about the customer: "Sometimes I feel lonely," Katheryn had said, quickly and quietly, after telling Peregrine about her "incredibly busy husband." Peregrine jotted down some notes and asked her to return in two weeks. "Oh, but I was hoping to wear this to an event on Saturday night!" the woman said, back to inhabiting her socialite's skin.

Peregrine felt a quick flash of irritation at the "right here right now" mentality but quickly reminded herself to place her own ego aside—a perfect lesson in patience for all involved. "Perfumes are a bit like people," she said. "They require time to blend and mature. We wouldn't want to rush that process."

That evening, Peregrine began to create the blend. She held the essence of Katheryn in her mind as she picked out the scents that would tell her story. Peregrine understood that she was a wealthy woman, used to getting what she wanted when she wanted it. She enjoyed reveling in the dramatic nonsense of the society world, similar to Alice at the Mad Hatter's tea party, but she felt alone in her wonder. She knew there were more holes to fall into, more paths to follow, and more stones to overturn, and couldn't bear the thought of leaving one unexplored. Worse, at the moment, she didn't have anyone with whom to chase the white rabbit. As she considered Katheryn's story—the one she spoke aloud and the one Peregrine sensed—she constructed the perfume's base, heart, and top notes. The base was mystical woods, strong enough to support Katheryn's beliefs but pliable enough to whisper magic from the treetops and into the wind like a puff of tobacco smoke sending desires to heaven. Peregrine added a heart of black pepper rose to spice up the soul and strengthen a love and a hat of delicate sweetness from neroli as she envisioned Katheryn chasing a white rabbit with all the innocent wonder of a little girl.

. . .

As time passed, Peregrine's fragrances—as well as Peregrine herself—gained more notoriety and a larger customer base. Most of her customers showered her with praise, and she deeply appreciated working with them, as they allowed her to live her dream. Some of them seemed to be in great emotional pain, and she couldn't help thinking of the path she had walked in her life and how different scents had helped her along the journey. She wanted to help these customers by supplying them with a way to create their own journey and travel where they wanted to go.

On her weekly phone call with Angela, Peregrine was recounting the story of one of her customers that day. "It was almost like looking into a mirror from fifteen years ago," she said. "I could tell she used to be vibrant and energetic, but now she's unhappy even as a newlywed. Granted, her marriage troubles were different from mine, but still, I wanted to—I intend to—create a perfume and a story to help her regain herself and then maintain her dreams and goals and never waver from them. I want her to live in the place of her heart that she's forgotten."

"It's still unbelievable to me what you're able to do through perfume," Angela said. "But you know you never can tell anyone much when they're in that place, right? I mean, remember your dad talking to you on your wedding day?"

Peregrine remembered standing in the back of church, so long ago, and how adamantly she'd refused her father's plea for her to leave, not marry Andrew, and wait until it was right. She simply hadn't been in a place where she was able to value her own life and happiness before someone else's. "I know, and I don't want to 'tell' them anything. I want them to come to their own realizations through experiencing an emotional antiphon. If I can create a perfume that takes people from their 'should-dos' to their 'want-tos,' that's the key. It's about using the power of their own emotions to influence their choices about the future."

Angela sounded impressed. "Preach it," she said. Then, changing the subject, she asked, "So how's it going with creating that pearl?"

Peregrine shrugged, though Angela couldn't see her, and looked out the window at dusk falling on the courtyard. Lush potted ferns, palms, oleanders, and gardenias swayed slightly in the evening breeze. Peregrine could just make out the soothing trickle from the fountain in the middle of the space.

"You know," she said, "I think it's actually going well. I know I create my own reality. I have to do the work."

However, Peregrine recognized that she had a lot of

work ahead of her to avoid becoming the type of close-minded, judgmental person that she once despised. She thought back to one Saturday, when she and Alice were driving to lunch. In passing, they saw a group of religious protesters holding picket signs outside a military funeral, their placards screaming pejorative, fundamental nonsense.

"Are they serious?" Alice cried. She looked at Peregrine with stunned eyes—she had never seen anything like this in Chicago. "What are these people thinking? How could they use someone's funeral as a platform for their cause? People are grieving in there!"

Peregrine felt the same rush of outrage as her daughter. "It's a terrible disrespect," she said. "But I also consciously try to feel empathy for those people picketing, as much as I disagree with what they believe, what they're doing, and how."

Alice's neck was craned, still staring at the picketers as they receded in the distance. "But how?" she asked. "How do you feel empathy for people who are clearly doing such a wrong thing?"

"They're coming from fear and misunderstanding," Peregrine said. She thought back to her own high school experiences here—recalling Todd and how others' fear and misunderstanding made him end his life. As always when she thought of him, she felt a swell of grief and anger in her chest but also one of gratitude for what he had inspired in her—a passionate refusal to simply fit in or to *give* in. And she thought of acupuncture school and all the lessons she'd learned about seeing people through pure love. She had realized there was more to people than what they presented, because she herself had hidden so much over the years. Everyone else had the right to do the same, and all she could do was try to remind herself that there was more, always more, than what the eye could perceive.

Alice looked at Peregrine, seeming lost in thought for a moment before she spoke. "I guess it just takes practice, huh?"

"That's for sure," Peregrine replied. "The trick is learning not to buy into the facades and judgments others put in the world; just look for the pure light within them. There is so much freedom when you let go of judgment. You don't have to be mad anymore or feel the weight of other people's baggage. You can just affect things around you as positively as possible and perhaps bring that positivity to others. You can live a beautiful life."

The two were quiet for the rest of their drive, each trying to shake off the effects of the protest and the funeral. Peregrine had to admit to herself that she wasn't having an easy time of it. Sometimes even her best intentions, her highest thoughts, didn't seem to be enough to counteract the lower-vibration feelings. In those times, she had to escape to somewhere else in her mind.

"Alice, do you remember when we lived in Colorado up on the side of the mountain?" At her daughter's nod, she continued. "Remember sitting out on the porch and watching the storms roll in from the west?"

Alice smiled. "Yeah."

Peregrine remembered sitting in silence on her porch, reflecting on the beauty surrounding her. *That* was meditation—quieting her mind and allowing herself to relax into the experience, to be present in the moment and not think about anything else. The beauty and majesty of the mountains allowed her to see how relative it all was. Peregrine was such a small part of this universe, yet so interconnected and important. The energy that she put out made a difference. In those tranquil moments when she witnessed the weather changes, watching nature and the changing leaves, the rising and setting of the sun, as she basked in silence—it was as if she sat on top of the world with the whole system beneath her. No matter what storm was being weathered below, it was always clear, sunny, and calm above.

"Being physically above the storms gave me so much clarity," Peregrine explained. "The key is to recognize the storms in our life and know that they always move on. The ability to stay connected to that calm above the storm can truly help us weather it."

Alice's troubled gaze seemed to clear a little. "Yeah, Mom," she said. "I think I know what you mean."

. . .

Over the next several months, Peregrine focused her energy on planning for the next phase in her life. Her dream of opening her own perfumery had only strengthened in the time she had been home, as had her vision for the store: the sumptuous jewel tones, the transformative energy, the seductive sense of falling into the rabbit hole, where all things were possible. Peregrine was thrumming with creative energy waiting to be manifested, and she knew that the only way to do that was to move from dreaming to action. So she used her growing reputation in the perfume industry to make connections with perfumers all over the country, attended every Chamber of Commerce meeting, volunteered with various community organizations, and worked hard to build authentic relationships and attract referrals. She started a bank account reserved strictly for her business, depositing a set percentage of her pay each month, and invested in her craft by traveling to Grasse, France, the home of perfumery, to take regular courses at the International Institute of Perfumery. On the limited time she had to herself on weekends, she scoured the city for spaces that matched her vision. With all her heart, she believed that within a year, she would be living her dream.

As Alice became increasingly independent—more like her mother—there were times when the house was empty and Peregrine's thoughts were able to wander away to a different dream. *I'd like to share my life with someone.* I don't *need* to, but I *want* to! For the first time, Peregrine felt whole, joyful, and confident that she wouldn't repeat the mistakes of her past in a new relationship. She knew now the kind of relationship she wanted—one of true partnership and respect, desire and sensuality, passion and drive, and love and admiration. She believed she was finally at a place in her life where true love was the only thing she could attract—and the only thing she would accept.

Though it was October and houses were already being decorated with crepe paper ghosts and flickering jack-o-lanterns, the morning was still fiercely humid when Peregrine dropped Alice off at school. "Don't forget," Alice said, giving Peregrine a quick peck on the cheek. "I've got tryouts for *Dracula* after school. I couldn't sleep at all last night because I was so excited. Rose said her mom can give me a ride home around seven."

"*Dracula*," Peregrine said, smiling. "That's one of my favorites. Good luck!"

As she drove to work, she let herself fall into a reverie, thinking of all the times she and Mimi had cuddled on the couch, watching their gothic movies. How fascinating—wondrous, almost—that her early education in peering behind the dark veil of what the eye could see led her on a path where she taught her daughter about pure white light. And now here Alice was, drawn to *Dracula* the way Peregrine had been as a girl. As she often did, Peregrine wondered who Alice would grow up to be.

Peregrine was the first at the perfumery that morning. She unlocked the door and went to the back room to drop off her bag, where she also slipped into her pristine white jacket. The store was dim and silent, almost mysterious in the morning light. The dark wooden floors bore the marks of many previous visitors, and dust hovered weightlessly in the rays of morning sunlight. As she straightened the glass bottles on the shelves, she returned to her earlier thoughts of wanting to share her life with someone amazing. Her heart felt wide open in her chest, welcoming, beckoning, and yet Peregrine knew it was also a heart filled with self-love. Her heart was ready to join with another. When the bell chimed, indicating that a customer had walked in, Peregrine jumped a little in surprise.

"I'm sorry," a man said, palms out in a conciliatory gesture. "I didn't mean to scare you. Are you open?"

Peregrine, a hand to her heart near the back wall of perfumes, nodded. She was struck by the elegant length of his fingers and his tall runner's physique. He was so good-looking and stylish, emanating a gentleness she could already feel. Flustered, Peregrine shook her head. "Well, no, we're not technically open for another half hour, but come in."

"Thanks," he said, his long-legged strides quickly closing the distance between them. "I'm on a flight back to New York in a couple of hours, and I was told I had to stop in here before I left."

Peregrine smiled, suffused with warmth, as she always was when a customer was a referral. "Well, let's hope we can make it worth your while, then. I'm Peregrine. What's your name?"

The man outstretched his hand. His crystal blue eyes met Peregrine's with an open, direct gaze. "I'm Christian."

For a moment, as he enclosed Peregrine's hand with his own, she felt light-headed. It was the exact opposite of the moment she'd met Brennan, sensing him to be an energy vampire. Christian's all-encompassing energy fulfilled Peregrine in an exquisitely strange way. Her heart pounded. Finally, she managed to breathe, "What can I do for you?"

"To tell you the truth," he said, "I'm not sure. A friend of mine said there was a woman—you, I suppose—who creates customized scents that are more than just fragrances." He shrugged, offering a wide, almost abashed grin. "She said you create stories . . . and that I should come find mine."

"I should hire your friend as my marketing director," Peregrine said with a laugh. She led him to a small, solid mahogany table, where they settled in opposite each other on the bench seats.

"Marketing director?" Christian asked. "Is this store yours, then? I was under the impression it had been here a very long time."

"It has," Peregrine said. "Almost a hundred years. But in the next year or so, I plan to open my own." She flushed, not sure why she was telling him this. "So, Christian, what do you do?"

"I work on Wall Street." He winced. "But don't hold that against me."

Peregrine laughed. "And what are you doing in New Orleans?"

Christian was quiet for a moment before answering, exploring her face with an intense, yet sweet, stare. Then he sighed. "I came to get away. Just for a long weekend. I've lived in New York for ten years and have worked on Wall Street for what feels like twice as long. I feel stuck on a path I forged years ago, when I was a different person, and I'm fairly convinced that life holds more for me than what I've always allowed myself to believe in. So I suppose you could say I'm contemplating diverging from my path."

Peregrine nodded. "Sometimes the path to getting what you want isn't straight and narrow," she said. "You might have to take some bends in the road—or, hell, make your own—but that just means life is presenting you with different opportunities for expansion." Peregrine smiled. "I've always loved the saying that sometimes we get lost on our path to fortuitously find treasure. The point is to enjoy the journey. You know?"

"Enjoy the journey," Christian said thoughtfully. "Have you ever heard the theory that life is like a diamond? Geometrically, I mean. When you're born, you're at the bottom tip, with everything stretching open before you. But by the time you're in the middle of your life, each choice you make takes you upward toward that narrow tip again."

"So each choice you make limits the numbers of choices you have left?" Peregrine asked with a laugh. "Well, that's depressing. I prefer to think of life more as a pearl. The pearl's luster—the most visible way to measure its quality—is more than just a surface reflection. It says something about the layers deep inside, reflecting and refracting light in a way that gives a sort of . . . infinite glow."

His eyes never left Peregrine's as she spoke. "So what's brought you here, Peregrine?"

She was startled. She was used to asking the questions, not being asked, and certainly not by someone who seemed so genuinely interested in the answer. He was leaning toward her slightly, his hands loosely laced on the table between them, and Peregrine had the sudden, strong desire to reach for those hands, stare into his eyes, and tell him everything—every mistake, every lesson, every flame in her that had dimmed, only to be stoked to burn brighter. Finally, she said:

"The pursuit of living beautifully."

Debrief

THE PEARLESCENT FLAME

YOU are iridescent! You can illuminate the world with all colors and hold all angles of perception. This is the level of superior transformation. In the pearlescent flame, we see the truth of all other flames and are able to manifest the truth of beauty from any flame source needed to transform. As the alchemist transmuting your life into an illuminated, iridescent, beautiful pearl through the power of each flame, you are the grand master of life, creating beauty of your mind, body, and spirit. You have, at your disposal, the tools to create beauty in your life. Know that each day of working toward creating unlimited potential is a process. Give yourself permission to revisit each flame; blow life into those flames that dim, and bask in the light of those that are strong and bright. You will create what you want in life when your flame lights guide you! Stay in alignment with yourself, and you will create the pearlescent flame. When the light from within you intertwines with the light shining upon you, you will be an exquisite wonder of nature.

ABOUT JESSICA PUCKETT

A lifelong lover of all things beautiful, Jessica Puckett is a board certified, licensed acupuncturist who also holds a master of science degree. She is the founder of a thriving health clinic in Memphis, Tennessee, where clients enjoy Jessica's expertise in facial rejuvenation and anti-aging treatments based in traditional Oriental medicine. Jessica is also the CEO of Perenelle, a luxury natural skincare line, and a partner in Karma Soma, a wellness coaching company that promotes self-care worldwide. In addition, she is a speaker, radio show host, and beauty/wellness coach. She has traveled the world studying beauty and wellness rituals and loves herbalism, essential oils, aromatherapy, and perfumes. Jessica's mission is to help people define, discover, and embrace their own authentic beauty. Currently, Jessica splits her time between her native Memphis and New York City.

Peregrine's story may or may not be inspired by Jessica's own transmutation.